Cardiovascular System

Roy D. Russ, PhD

Associate Professor of Pharmacology
Division of Basic Medical Sciences
Mercer University School of Medicine
Macon, Georgia

UK edition authors
Toby Fagan and Romeshan Sunthareswaran

UK series editor
Daniel Horton-Szar

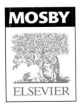

MOSBY

ELSEVIER

MOSBY
ELSEVIER

1600 John F. Kennedy Boulevard
Suite 1800
Philadelphia, PA 19103-2899

CRASH COURSE: CARDIOVASCULAR SYSTEM   ISBN-13: 978-0-323-04345-8
Copyright © 2006 by Mosby, Inc., an affiliate of Elsevier Inc.   ISBN-10: 0-323-04345-3

Adapted from Crash Course Cardiovascular System 2e by Toby Fagan, ISBN 0-7234-3249-X.
© 2002, Elsevier Science Limited. All rights reserved.

The rights of Toby Fagan to be identified as the author of this work have been asserted by him in accordance with the Copyright Designs and Patents Act, 1988.

Library of Congress Cataloging-in-Publication Data

Russ, Roy D.
    Crash course: cardiovascular system/Roy D. Russ.—1st ed.
        p. ; cm.—(Crash course)
    Includes index.
    ISBN 0-323-04345-3
    1. Cardiovascular system.   I. Title: Cardiovascular system.   II. Title.   III. Series.
    [DNLM: 1. Cardiovascular System.   2. Cardiovascular Diseases.   3. Cardiovascular Physiology.
    WG 100 R958c 2006]
    QP102.R875 2006
    612.1—dc22   2005057653

Commissioning Editor: Alex Stibbe
Developmental Editor: Stan Ward
Project Manager: David Saltzberg
Design: Andy Chapman
Cover Design: Antbits Illustration
Illustration Manager: Mick Ruddy

Printed in China.

Last digit is the print number:
9 8 7 6 5 4 3 2 1

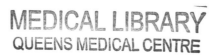

Working together to grow
libraries in developing countries

www.elsevier.com | www.bookaid.org | www.sabre.org

ELSEVIER   BOOK AID International   Sabre Foundation

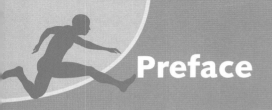

Preface

Medicine in general and cardiovascular medicine in particular are fields at a crossroad. We are on the verge of exciting discoveries that are likely to change our understanding of the fundamental processes underlying current diagnosis and treatment. At the same time, we must be very careful not to lose sight of the principles and ideas that have served us so well in the past.

My goal in this edition is to make the cardiovascular system, with all its pumps, valves, pipes, and gurgles, a bit more understandable. It is not meant to be an exhaustive text; rather, it is intended to reinforce important concepts. If you come across a section that is foreign to you, then I would refer you to any number of excellent textbooks. Similarly, if your main textbook sometimes seems a bit too abstract, I hope this text will make the information more palatable. My other hope is that *Crash Course: Cardiovascular System* will serve as a valuable review for the national board exams. If it is useful in your clerkships, that would be great as well.

Preparing this text has been a fun and exciting learning experience for me, and I hope it will prove to be useful for you. Good luck in your studies. I wish you a long and enjoyable career.

Roy D. Russ, PhD

Acknowledgments

Thanks to the authors of the UK editions, Toby Fagan and Romeshan Sunthareswaran, as well as the series editor, Daniel Horton-Szar.

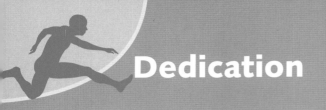

Dedication

To
my students, for challenging me
my colleagues, for holding me accountable
my extended family, for being there
my parents, for setting the example
my children, for inspiring me
Deborah, for everything.

Contents

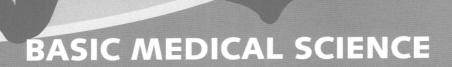

BASIC MEDICAL SCIENCE

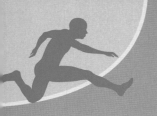

1. Overview of the Cardiovascular System

Why do we need a cardiovascular system?

The cardiovascular system serves to provide rapid transport of nutrients around the body and rapid removal of waste products. In smaller, less complex organisms, there is no such system because they can supply their needs by simple diffusion. The human body, however, is too large for simple diffusion to be effective. Evolution of the cardiovascular system provided a means of aiding the diffusion process, which allowed for the development of larger organisms.

The cardiovascular system allows nutrients to do the following:
- Diffuse into the system at their source (e.g., oxygen from the lungs).
- Travel long distances quickly.
- Diffuse into tissues where they are needed (e.g., oxygen to working muscle).

This process is called convective transport, and it requires energy. The heart supplies this energy, and the blood vessels provide the circuit for transport of nutrients and waste products. Because the cardiovascular system serves a large, multicellular organism, the functions of the system must rely on a medium for transport of nutrients and waste products. The blood serves as this medium. Blood is composed of cells (primarily red blood cells) and plasma (water, proteins, etc.), both of which serve as the transport medium for various substances.

Functions of the cardiovascular system

The main functions of the cardiovascular system are:
- Rapid transport of nutrients (oxygen, amino acids, glucose, fatty acids, water, etc.) and waste products (carbon dioxide, urea, creatinine, etc.).
- Hormonal control, by transporting hormones to their target organs and by secreting its own hormones (e.g., atrial natriuretic peptide).
- Temperature regulation, by controlling heat distribution between the body core and the skin.
- Reproduction, by producing erection of the penis.
- Host defense, transporting immune cells, antigens, and other mediators (e.g., antibody).

The heart and circulation

The heart is a double pump. It consists of two muscular pumps (the left and right ventricles). Each pump has its own reservoir (the left and right atrium).

The two pumps each serve a different circulation. A typical blood cell flows first in one circulation and then moves into the other.

The right ventricle is the pump for the pulmonary circulation. Blood is pumped into the lungs, where it acquires oxygen and loses carbon dioxide; it then returns to the left atrium of the heart. This blood then enters the left ventricle.

The left ventricle is the pump for the systemic circulation. Blood is pumped from the left ventricle to the rest of the body. In the tissues of the body, nutrients and waste products are exchanged. Blood (which now carries less oxygen and more carbon dioxide) returns to the right atrium and then into the right ventricle.

The pulmonary circulation is usually of lower pressure than the systemic circulation, because the pulmonary circulation has lower vascular resistance.

The two circulations operate simultaneously, with blood constantly flowing in each circulation. They can be thought of as being in series, with each circulation supplied by a different pump. This one-way, circular pathway for blood is brought about partly by the presence of valves in the heart and veins (Fig. 1.1).

The circulatory system is made up of arteries, veins, capillaries, and lymphatic vessels.
- Arteries transport blood from the heart to the body tissues.
- Capillaries are where diffusion of nutrients and waste products take place.
- Veins return blood from the tissues to the heart.
- Lymphatic vessels return to the blood any excess water and nutrients that have diffused out of the capillaries.

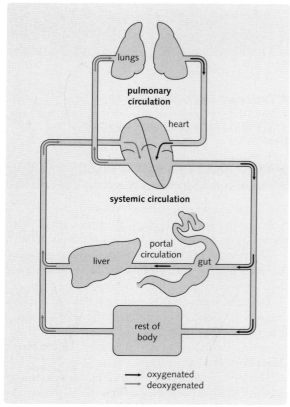

Fig. 1.1 Systemic and pulmonary circulations. Unidirectional flow is maintained by valves in the heart and the pressure difference between the arterial and venous systems. It is aided by valves in the venous system.

The entire cardiac output of the right ventricle passes through the lungs. The cardiac output of the left ventricle passes into the aorta, and it is distributed to various organs and tissues according to their metabolic requirements or particular functions (e.g., skeletal muscle gets a larger blood supply during exercise than at rest; the kidney receives a relatively high percentage [20%] of cardiac output so that its excretory function can be maintained). This distribution can be changed to meet the varying demands of different tissues (e.g., after eating, blood flow to the intestines increases to allow for nutrient absorption).

Blood is driven along the vessels by pressure. This pressure, which is produced by the ejection of blood from the ventricles, is highest in the aorta (about 120 mmHg above atmospheric pressure) and lowest in the great veins (almost atmospheric). It is this pressure difference that moves blood through the arterial tree, through the capillaries, and into the veins. In the veins, the movement of blood is driven by a pressure gradient and aided by one-way valves. Note that pressure gradients provide the "driving force" for blood flow but do not determine the direction of blood flow. This vital function is determined by resistance. This will be discussed later in greater detail.

Arterial blood flow is pulsatile, with a higher pressure during systole than diastole.

The amount of blood ejected from one ventricle during a 1-minute period is called the cardiac output. The cardiac output of each ventricle is equal overall, but there may be occasional beat-by-beat variation.

Systole is when the two ventricles contract nearly simultaneously, whereas diastole is when the two ventricles relax together.

- What are the functions of the cardiovascular system?
- How are the two circulations organized?
- What are some factors that might alter the flow and distribution of blood through the two circulations?

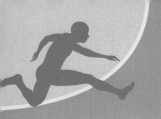

Organization of cardiac tissue

Anatomy of the heart and great vessels

Mediastinum

This is the space between the two lungs and pleurae. It contains all the structures of the chest except the lungs and pleurae (Figs. 2.1 and 2.2).

The mediastinum extends from the superior thoracic aperture to the diaphragm and from the sternum to the vertebrae. The structures in the mediastinum are surrounded by loose connective tissue, nerves, blood, and lymph vessels. It can accommodate movement and volume changes.

The mediastinum is often subdivided into superior and inferior parts. The superior part contains:
- Anteriorly, the thymus.
- In the middle, the heart and pericardium, great arteries, phrenic nerve, and main bronchi.
- Posteriorly, esophagus, trachea, and thoracic duct.

Inferiorly, the mediastinum contains:
- Anteriorly, the thymus.
- In the middle, the heart and pericardium, great arteries, phrenic nerve, and main bronchi.

- Posteriorly, the esophagus and thoracic aorta.

The heart is in the middle mediastinum, and it has the following relations:
- Superiorly, the great vessels and bronchi.
- Inferiorly, the diaphragm.
- Laterally, the pleurae and lungs.

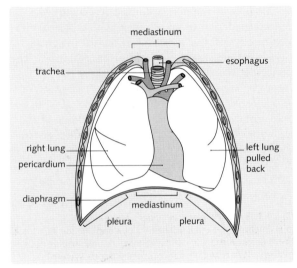

Fig. 2.1 Anterior view of the mediastinum.

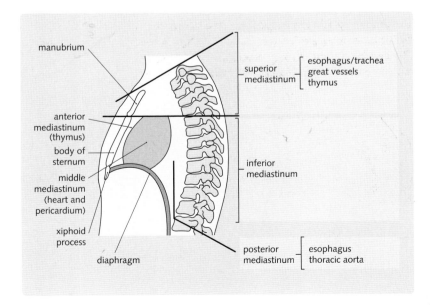

Fig. 2.2 Lateral view of the mediastinum.

- Anteriorly, the thymus.
- Posteriorly, the esophagus.

Pericardium

The pericardium is a fibroserous sac, consisting of tough fibrous tissue, enclosing the heart. Picture your fist pushed into a balloon until it is completely surround by rubber. The heart sits inside the pericardium in a similar fashion. The outer surface of the heart and the inner surface of pericardium are covered with transparent layers of serous pericardium. Between these layers, there is pericardial fluid, secreted by the serous pericardium.

The base of the pericardium is fused with the central tendon of the diaphragm. The pericardium is also fused with the tunica adventitia of the great vessels entering and leaving the heart. Anteriorly, the pericardium is joined to the sternum by the sternopericardial ligaments.

There are two sinuses (pouches or pockets) in the pericardium; they are formed by the folding of the embryological heart, which produces reflections in the pericardium:

- The transverse pericardial sinus is a recess within the pericardium, posterior to the aorta and pulmonary trunk and anterior to the superior vena cava.

- The oblique pericardial sinus is a blind recess formed by the inferior vena cava and pulmonary veins.

External structure of the heart

The heart lies obliquely about two thirds to the left and one third to the right of the median plane (Figs. 2.3–2.5). It has the following surfaces:

- The base of the heart is located posteriorly and formed mainly by the left atrium.
- The apex of the heart is formed by the left ventricle and is posterior to the fifth intercostal space.
- The sternocostal surface of the heart is formed mainly by the right ventricle.
- The diaphragmatic surface is formed mainly by the left ventricle and part of the right ventricle.
- The pulmonary surface is mainly formed by the left ventricle.

The heart borders of the anterior surface are as follows:

- Right: right atrium.
- Left: left ventricle and left auricle.
- Inferior: right ventricle mainly and part of left ventricle.
- Superior: right and left auricles.

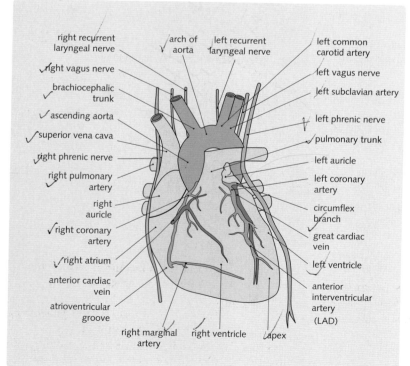

Fig. 2.3 Sternocostal external view of the heart.

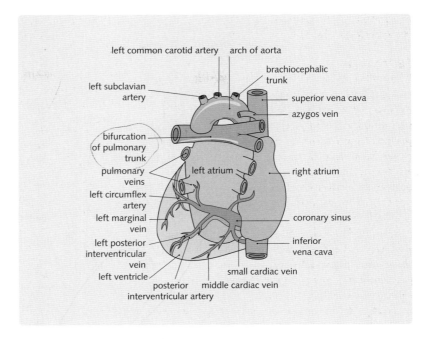

Fig. 2.4 Posteroinferior external view of the heart.

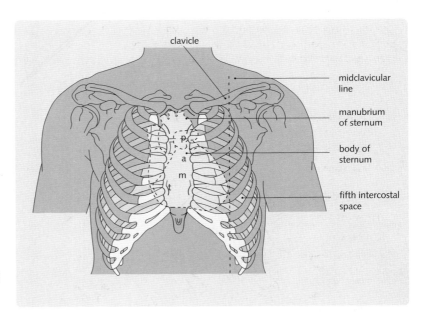

Fig. 2.5 Surface markings of the heart (a, aortic valve; m, mitral valve; p, pulmonic valve; t, tricuspid valve). See Fig. 7.10 for auscultatory areas.

Internal structure of the heart

The internal structure of the heart is shown in Fig. 2.6. The right atrium contains the orifices, or openings, of the superior and inferior venae cavae and coronary sinus.

The right ventricle is separated from the right atrium by the tricuspid (three cusps) valve. The right ventricle is separated from its outflow tract (the pulmonary trunk) by the pulmonic valve. This has three semilunar valve cusps.

The left atrium has the orifices of four pulmonary veins in its posterior wall. The left atrium is separated from the left ventricle by the mitral (two cusps) valve. The left ventricle is separated from its

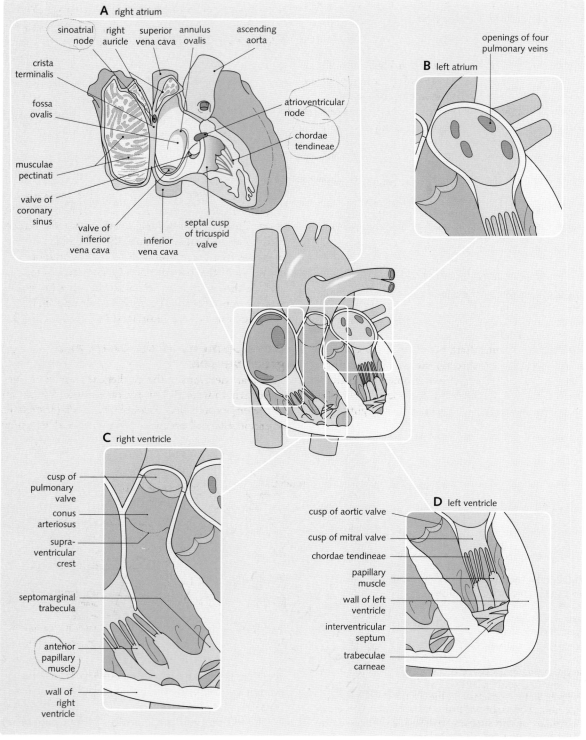

Fig. 2.6 Internal structure of the four chambers of the heart. A. Right atrium. B. Left atrium. C. Right ventricle. D. Left ventricle.

outflow tract (the aorta) by the aortic valve. This also has three semilunar valve cusps.

Coronary arteries

The coronary arteries are shown in Figs. 2.7 and 2.8.

The left coronary artery arises from the root of the aorta just past the left anterior cusp of the aortic valve. The right coronary artery arises from the right anterior aortic sinus just above the right anterior cusp of the aortic valve.

> Remember that many surgeons still use the term left anterior descending coronary artery (LAD) when referring to the anterior interventricular artery (AIA). The boards should use the latter, more current term, but you should know both.

Coronary veins

The coronary veins drain mainly into the coronary sinus, which drains directly into the right atrium (Figs. 2.9 and 2.10). There are some small veins that drain directly into the heart chambers. Generally, these "thebesian veins" drain into the right side of the heart.

> Note that a small amount of venous blood empties directly into the RV without going through the lungs. This slightly lowers oxygen tension in RV blood compared with venous pulmonary blood. This concept is commonly tested by the United States Medical Licensing Examination.

Great vessels

The "great vessels" is the term used to denote the large arteries and veins that are directly related to the heart. The great arteries include the pulmonary trunk and the aorta (and sometimes its three main branches: the brachiocephalic, the left common carotid, and the left subclavian). The great veins include the pulmonary veins and the superior and inferior venae cavae. The great vessels and their thoracic branches are illustrated in Figs. 2.11–2.13.

Development of the heart and great vessels

The heart develops in the cardiogenic region of the mesoderm in week 3. This region is at the cranial end of the embryonic disc. Angioblastic cords (aggregates of endothelial cell precursors) develop, and here they

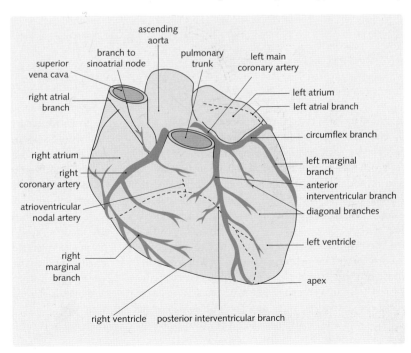

Fig. 2.7 Anterior surface of the heart showing coronary arteries. The left coronary artery has two terminal branches: the anterior interventricular branch (also called the left anterior descending [LAD]) and the circumflex branch. The anterior interventricular branch supplies both ventricles and the interventricular septum. The circumflex branch supplies the left atrium and the inferior part of the left ventricle. The right coronary artery supplies the sinoatrial (SA) node via the right atrial branch.

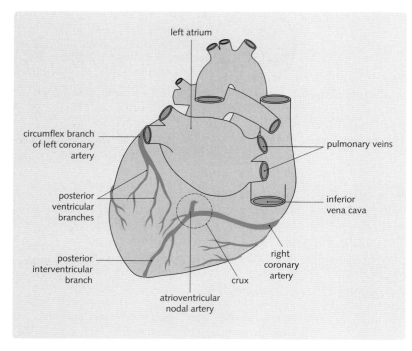

Fig. 2.8 Posteroinferior surface of the heart showing coronary arteries. The right coronary artery gives off a right marginal branch (see Fig. 2.7) and a large posterior interventricular branch. Near the apex, the posterior interventricular branch may anastomose with the anterior interventricular branch of the left coronary artery. The right coronary artery mainly supplies the right atrium, right ventricle, and interventricular septum. It may also supply part of the left atrium and left ventricle. The nodal branch supplies the atrioventricular (AV) node.

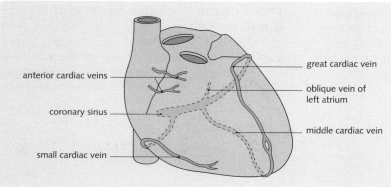

Fig. 2.9 Anterior view of the heart showing coronary veins.

coalesce to form two lateral endocardial tubes. During week 4, these tubes fuse together to form the primitive heart tube, and the heart begins to pump (Fig. 2.14).

From weeks 5 to 8, the primitive heart tube folds and remodels to form the four-chambered heart. Initially, the primitive heart tube develops a series of expansions separated by shallow sulci (infoldings, Fig. 2.15).

The primitive atrium will give rise to parts of both future atria. The primitive ventricle will make up most of the left ventricle. The bulbus cordis will form the right ventricle. The truncus arteriosus will form the ascending aorta and the pulmonary trunk.

Venous blood initially enters the sinus horns of the sinus venosus from the cardinal veins (branches

of the umbilical vein). Within the next few weeks, the whole systemic venous return is shifted to the right sinus horn through the newly formed superior and inferior venae cavae. The left sinus horn becomes the coronary sinus, which drains the myocardium.

The right sinus horn and part of the venae cavae are incorporated into the growing right atrium to form the posterior wall (Fig. 2.16). This process occurs by intussusception (imagine stretching the opening of a tubular elastic bandage—as the opening widens, the bandage shortens). This gives the smooth wall of the bulk of the atrium, while the original, trabeculated right half of the atrium forms the right auricle.

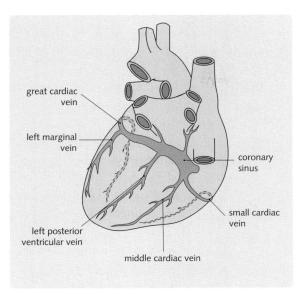

Fig. 2.10 Posteroinferior view of the heart showing coronary veins.

The original left half of the primitive atrium grows a pulmonary vein, which branches as it moves towards the lungs to form the pulmonary venous system. Eventually, the trunk of the pulmonary vein (which has grown from the primitive atrium) is incorporated (again by intussusception) to form most of the left atrium. As this process continues, more of the pulmonary venous system is gradually incorporated into the atrium. Initially, there is only one orifice, but the process continues until the second bifurcation is reached, and four orifices result. Again, the original, trabeculated atrial wall forms the left auricle.

A pair of valves (the venous valves) develop at the orifices of the venae cavae and the coronary sinus. Superior to these orifices, the valves fuse to form a transient septum spurium. The left valve eventually becomes part of the septum secundum. The right valve develops into the valves of the inferior vena cava and the coronary sinus.

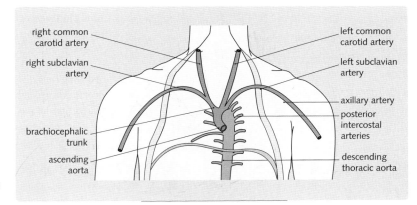

Fig. 2.11 The thoracic aorta and its branches.

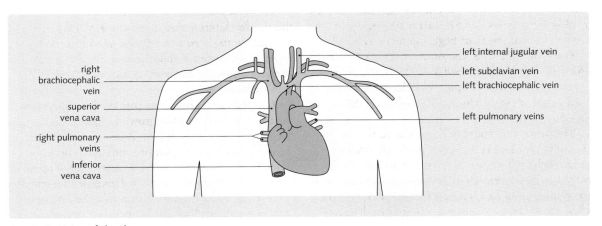

Fig. 2.12 Veins of the thorax.

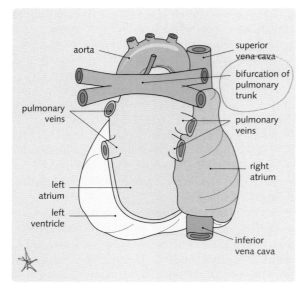

Fig. 2.13 Pulmonary vessels.

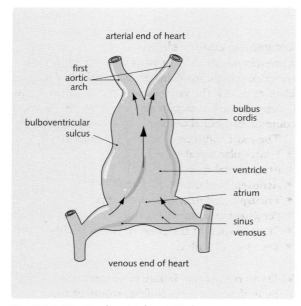

Fig. 2.14 Primitive heart tube at 21 days.

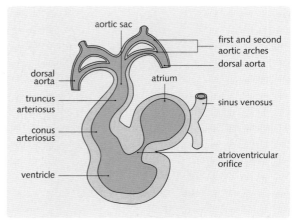

Fig. 2.15 Primitive heart tube as it folds and expands.

between the atria. The septum primum grows downward from the superior posterior wall. The foramen (ostium primum) it creates narrows as the septum grows.

The endocardium around the atrioventricular canal (between the atria and the ventricles) grows to form four expansions. These are the left, right, superior, and inferior endocardial cushions.

At the end of week 6, the superior and inferior cushions meet and fuse together to form the septum intermedium, which creates the left and right atrioventricular canals (Fig. 2.18). At the same time, the edge of the septum primum fuses with the septum intermedium, closing the ostium primum. However, before complete closure of the ostium primum, cell death in the superior part of the septum primum creates small openings, which join together to form the ostium secundum. This maintains the shunt between the two atria.

While the septum primum is growing, a thicker septum secundum also starts to form. This septum secundum does not meet the septum intermedium, leaving an opening called the foramen ovale near the floor of the right atrium.

Blood now has to shunt from the right to the left atrium through the two staggered openings in the septum, the foramen ovale and the ostium secundum (Fig. 2.19). At birth, the pressure rises in the left atrium, pushing the septum primum against the septum secundum, effectively closing the foramen ovale. Over time, the two septa are fused together to abolish any communication between the two atria.

During weeks 5–6, the atrioventricular valves develop. The heart undergoes changes that bring the

A ridge of tissue, the crista terminalis, forms superior to the right valve marking the edge of the right auricle, and this will eventually form part of the conduction pathway from the sinoatrial node to the atrioventricular node.

In weeks 5–6, the septum primum and the septum secundum grow to separate the right and left atria (Fig. 2.17). These septa are incomplete and leave two openings (foramina or ostia) that allow blood to move

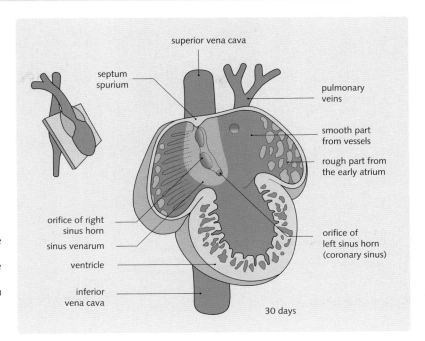

Fig. 2.16 Initial differentiation of the primitive atrium. The primitive atrium derives from two tissues: the rough part from early atrial tissue; the smooth part from venous tissue that spreads as the veins "push" into the developing atrium (redrawn from *Human Embryology*, 2nd ed. by Larsen WJ, New York, Churchill Livingstone, 1997).

atria and ventricles into their correct positions and align the outflow tracts with the ventricles.

The inferior part of the bulboventricular sulcus grows into the muscular ventricular septum. Growth stops in week 7, which allows for the left outflow tract to develop. This leaves an interventricular foramen.

In weeks 7–8, the truncus arteriosus (the common outflow tract of the heart) is divided in two by a spiral process of central septation, which results in the formation of the aorta and pulmonary trunk. This septum is called the truncoconal septum.

This septum also grows into the ventricles, and it forms the membranous ventricular septum, which joins the muscular ventricular septum. This completes the septation of the ventricles.

Swellings develop at the inferior end of the truncus arteriosus, and these give rise to the semilunar arterial valves.

There are many difficult terms in embryology. Try to understand them by considering what process the term describes. For example, the septum primum is the first (primus means first in Latin) septum to form, and septum secundum is the second septum to form.

Congenital abnormalities

The embryologic development of the heart is a complex process involving many coordinated steps. Defects arise if the process does not occur correctly. Congenital cardiovascular abnormalities are the most common congenital defects in live births.

The most common abnormalities include:
- Ventricular septal defect (VSD).
- Atrial septal defect (ASD).
- Atrioventricular septal defect (AVSD).
- Tricuspid and mitral valve defects.
- Persistent truncus arteriosus.
- Transposition of the great arteries (TGA).
- Tetralogy of Fallot.

VSD can result from failure of the muscular and membranous septa to fuse, failure of the endocardial cushions to fuse (also causes AVSD), or perforation of the muscular septum during development.

There are many types of ASD, including patent foramen ovale and secundum ASD. Patent foramen ovale occurs when the septum primum and septum secundum fail to fuse together at birth, allowing blood to shunt across. A secundum ASD results when the septum secundum fails to grow completely and therefore does not cover the ostium secundum. Thus, when the septum primum and secundum fuse, a hole is still present.

13

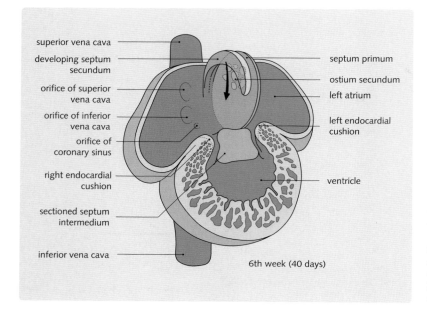

superior vena cava
developing septum secundum
orifice of superior vena cava
orifice of inferior vena cava
orifice of coronary sinus
right endocardial cushion
sectioned septum intermedium
inferior vena cava

septum primum
ostium secundum
left atrium
left endocardial cushion
ventricle

6th week (40 days)

Fig. 2.17 Initial septation of the atria. The septum primum forms at day 33 and eventually leaves a hole (the ostium secundum). The septum secundum develops later at day 40 and is deficient at the foramen ovale (redrawn from *Human Embryology*, 2nd ed. by Larsen WJ, New York, Churchill Livingstone, 1997).

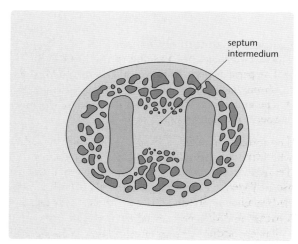

septum intermedium

Fig. 2.18 Cross-section of heart at the atrioventricular level at the end of week 6. The superior and inferior endocardial cushions fuse to form the septum intermedium. This produces two atrioventricular canals.

AVSD can result from failure of the superior and inferior endocardial cushions to fuse. Tricuspid and mitral valve defects result from errors in the development of the valves from the ventricular wall.

In persistent truncus arteriosus, the truncoconal septum fails to form, leading to a common outflow tract for both ventricles. There is also a VSD.

TGA occurs when the truncoconal septum develops, but it does not spiral. The left ventricle pumps blood into the pulmonary trunk, and the right ventricle pumps blood into the aorta. There is usually also a patent foramen ovale or patent ductus arteriosus to allow blood to mix.

Tetralogy of Fallot is a combination of pulmonary stenosis, right ventricular hypertrophy, overriding aorta, and VSD. The primary problem is failure of the outflow regions to align properly. This causes stenosis around the subpulmonary outlet, which leads to right ventricular hypertrophy. A VSD also occurs because of malalignment, since fusion between the membranous and muscular septum cannot take place. The abnormality also displaces the aorta to the right, causing it to override the interventricular septum and receive output from both the left and right ventricles.

These congenital abnormalities are illustrated and further discussed in Chapter 5, beginning on p. 108.

Tissue layers of the heart and pericardium

The heart contains three layers (Fig. 2.20):
• Pericardium.
• Myocardium.
• Endocardium.

Pericardium

The pericardium consists of an outer fibrous pericardial sac, enclosing the whole heart, and an inner double layer of flat mesothelial cells, called the serous pericardium.

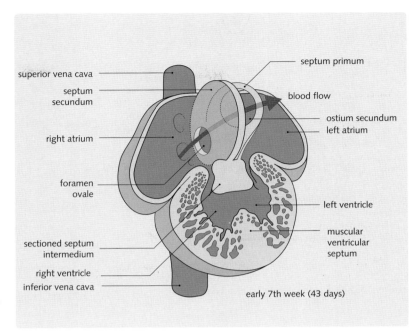

Fig. 2.19 Completed septation of the atria. The septum primum is deficient superiorly at the ostium secundum. The septum secundum is deficient inferiorly at the foramen ovale. Blood shunts from the right atrium through these two holes in the septa to the left atrium. In this way, blood bypasses the lungs in the fetal circulation. As these two openings are staggered, fusion of the septum primum and secundum will abolish any shunt between the atria (redrawn from *Human Embryology*, 2nd ed. by Larsen WJ, New York, Churchill Livingstone, 1997).

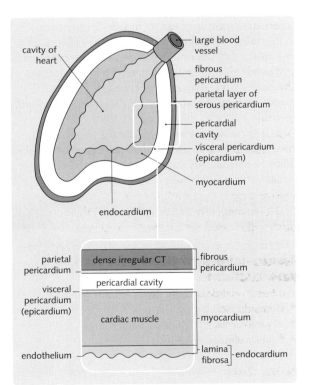

Fig. 2.20 Tissue layers of the heart and pericardium (CT, connective tissue).

The two layers of the serous pericardium are:
- The parietal pericardium, which is attached to the fibrous sac.
- The visceral pericardium (or epicardium), which covers the heart's outer surface.

The serous pericardium produces pericardial fluid, which consists primarily of a plasma ultrafiltrate. The pericardial cavity formed by the parietal and visceral layers contains approximately 50 mL of this fluid in a normal individual. Its primary function is lubrication of the pericardial membranes.

The epicardium's thin internal layer of connective tissue contains adipose tissue, nerves, and the coronary arteries and veins.

Myocardium

Myocardium is the thickest layer of the heart, and it consists of cardiac muscle cells. The thickness and cell diameter are greatest in the left ventricle and thinnest in the atria. All the muscle layers attach to the heart skeleton, which provides a base for contraction.

In addition to its role in contraction, the atrial myocardium also participates in cardiovascular regulation by secreting atrial natriuretic peptide (ANP). This peptide is secreted during hypervolemia

15

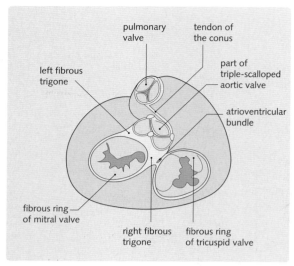

Fig. 2.21 Superior view of the heart skeleton. Vessels and external muscle layers have been removed.

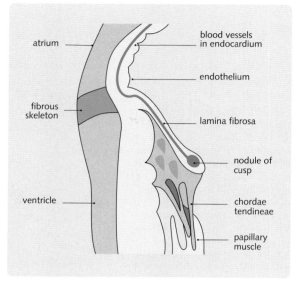

Fig. 2.22 Structure of a heart valve.

and signals the kidneys to increase salt and water excretion.

Endocardium

The endocardial layer consists of two layers: an innermost single layer of endothelial cells and a subendothelial layer of connective tissue called the lamina fibrosa. The lamina fibrosa contains nerves, veins, and specialized conductive cells called Purkinje fibers.

Heart skeleton

The heart skeleton consists of fibrotendinous (fibrocollagenous) rings of dense connective tissue that encircle the base of the aorta and pulmonary trunk and the atrioventricular openings (Fig. 2.21). The heart valves and cardiac muscle attach to these rings. The heart skeleton anchors the heart for contraction.

The skeleton also electrically insulates the atria from the ventricles. The atrioventricular node forms the only conduction pathway through the skeleton and is, therefore, the only electrical link between the atria and the ventricles.

Valves

The heart valves are avascular (i.e., they have no blood supply) (Fig. 2.22). This is important if bacteria invade the valves, because there is little immune reaction, and infective endocarditis often results.

Myocardium
Cardiac myocytes

There are three types of myocytes—cardiac muscle cells, nodal cells, and conduction fibers (Fig. 2.23):
- Cardiac muscle cells are the main contractile cells.
- Nodal cells generate cardiac electrical impulses.
- Conduction (Purkinje) fibers allow fast conduction of action potentials around the heart.

The myocardium is innervated by autonomic (sympathetic and parasympathetic) nerves controlled from the brainstem.

Cellular physiology of the heart

Ultrastructure of the typical myocyte

The typical cardiac myocyte (Fig. 2.24) has the following features:
- Length of 50–100 μm (shorter than skeletal muscle fibers).
- Diameter of 10–20 μm.
- Single, central nucleus.
- Branched structure.
- Attached to neighboring cells via intercalated disks at the branch points. These cell junctions consist of desmosomes (which hold the cells together via proteoglycan bridges) and gap junctions (which allow electrical conductivity).

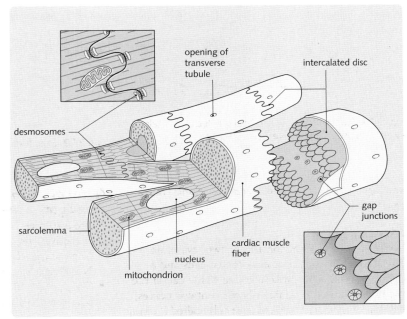

Fig. 2.23 Types of myocytes. The action potential (AP) is initiated in the nodal cells. It is then rapidly conducted through the Purkinje fibers to the work myocytes where contraction occurs.

Fig. 2.24 Cardiac myocyte arrangement. Myocytes are branched, and they attach to each other through desmosomes to form muscle fibers. Gap junctions enable rapid electrical conductivity between cells. There is an extensive sarcoplasmic reticulum, which is the internal Ca^{2+} store. The contractile elements within each cell produce characteristic bands and lines. In between each myofibril unit, there are rows of mitochondria. Accompanying blood vessels and connective tissue lie alongside each muscle fiber (redrawn with permission from *Principles of Anatomy and Physiology*, 9th ed. by Tortora GJ, Grabowski SR, New York, John Wiley & Sons, 2000).

- Many mitochondria arranged in rows between the intracellular myofibrils.
- T (transverse) tubules organized in dyads with cisternae of sarcoplasmic reticulum (Fig. 2.25), which enable rapid electrical conduction deep into the cell, activating the whole contractile apparatus simultaneously.
- Extensive sarcoplasmic reticulum, which stores Ca^{2+} ions.

Each myocyte contains many myofibril-like units (similar to the myofibrils of skeletal muscle) (see Fig. 2.25).

These myofibril-like units are made up of many sarcomeres attached end-to-end and collected into a bundle.

A sarcomere is the basic contractile unit. It is composed of two bands, the A band and the I band, between two Z lines.

The A (anisotropic) band is made up of thick myosin filaments and some interdigitating actin filaments.

The I (isotropic) band is made up of thin actin filaments that do not overlap with myosin filaments. Troponin and tropomyosin are also contained in the thin filaments.

The Z line is a dark-staining structure containing α-actinin protein that provides attachment for the thin filaments.

Excitation and action potentials
Resting membrane potential
The resting membrane potential of a cardiac cell is approximately –80 mV (Fig. 2.26). This value is determined by the distribution of ions across the membrane and the differential permeability of the membrane. In cardiac myocytes, it is the K$^+$ gradient

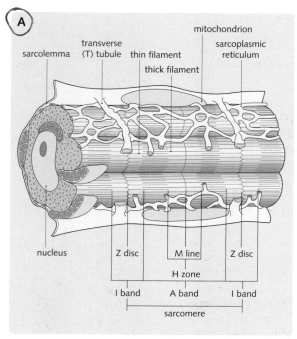

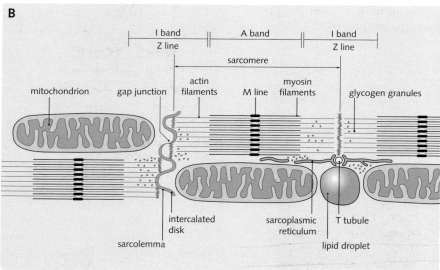

Fig. 2.25 Electronmicrographic appearance of cardiac muscle. A. Each myocyte has rows of mitochondria in between myofibril-like units. There is also an extensive sarcoplasmic reticulum and T tubule system (redrawn from *Gray's Anatomy*, 37th ed. by Williams PL [ed], New York, Churchill Livingstone, 1989). B. Close-up of a myofibril-like unit shows the following bands: A band, myosin with some actin; I band, actin; Z line, attachment point for actin (redrawn from *Human Physiology* by Davies A, Blakeley AGH, Kidd C, New York, Churchill Livingstone, 2001).

that is the major determinant of the resting membrane potential. The potential can be predicted using the Nernst equation:

$$E_K = -65 \log \left(\frac{[K^+]_{out}}{[K^+]_{in}} \right)$$

There is a discrepancy between the predicted value and the actual value. This is due to the leakage of small numbers of Na^+ ions inward and K^+ ions outward across the membrane and the action of the enzyme Na^+/K^+ ATPase, which actively pumps Na^+ out of and K^+ into the cells. This pump supplies the driving force for the generation of a resting membrane potential.

Cardiac glycosides, such as digitalis, inhibit the Na^+/K^+ ATPase pump, partially lowering the transmembrane Na^+ gradient.

Action potential

The cardiac action potential (Fig. 2.27) lasts about 300 ms in cardiac muscle cells. The arrival of an action potential from an adjacent cell causes the cell membrane to depolarize to threshold. Na^+ channels then open rapidly, generating the fast upstroke. This subsequently opens Ca^{2+} channels, and this produces the plateau phase. K^+ channels are also opened, which eventually leads to repolarization. The late part of the plateau phase is sustained in part by the action of the Na^+–Ca^{2+} exchanger. Nerve action potentials, in contrast to the cardiac action potential, last only 3 ms, and they do not have a plateau phase.

Ca^{2+} ions flow into the cell during the plateau phase (Fig. 2.28); thus, it helps determine the strength of contraction. In addition, the cell is refractory to further stimulation during this phase, which prevents tetonic contractions.

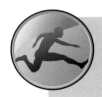

Make sure you can draw a typical cardiac action potential and explain how it is brought about. This is the basis for many board questions.

Calcium is the key ion in muscles. Changing its concentration is the basis of many of the actions of the nervous system, hormones, and some drugs that act on the heart and vessels (e.g., norepinehrine from sympathetic nerves increases intracellular Ca^{2+} and increases contractile force).

Na^+ channels are blocked by tetrodotoxin, leading to a slower upstroke and prolonged action potential.

Ca^{2+} channels are blocked by verapamil, leading to a shorter plateau phase and action potential, which decreases contractility. They are opened by

Ion concentrations			
Ion	Plasma concentration (mmol/L)	Intracellular concentration (mmol/L)	Equilibrium potential (mV)
Na^+	135–145	10	70
K^+	3.5–5.0	135	−94
Cl^-	120	30	−36

Fig. 2.26 Intracellular and extracellular ionic concentrations.

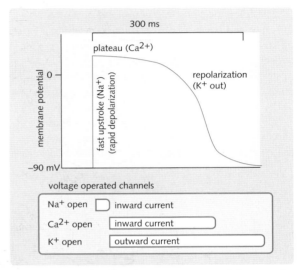

Fig. 2.27 Diagram of cardiac action potential showing the timing of ionic current flow.

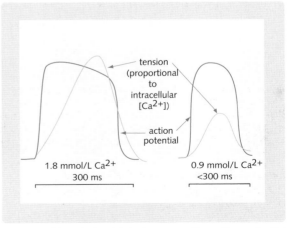

Fig. 2.28 The relationship between cardiac action potential and extracellular Ca^{2+} concentration.

epinephrine, enhancing the plateau phase and increasing contractility.

K$^+$ channels are blocked by a number of antiarrhythmic agents, prolonging repolarization and potentially leading to life-threatening complications.

Variation in action potential
Sinoatrial node

The sinoatrial (SA) node is located in the posterior wall of the right atrium. It is the cardiac pacemaker and is responsible for initiating the depolarization and, therefore, contraction of the whole heart.

The SA node's resting membrane potential is unstable and has a tendency to become more positive. When it reaches a threshold value, it triggers off an action potential (Fig. 2.29). The upstroke of the action potential is slow because it is mediated by a Ca^{2+} current and not a Na$^+$ current, as in the fast upstrokes of ventricular myocytes.

The SA node is controlled by the autonomic nervous system. Sympathetic stimulation increases the rate of decay of the resting membrane potential,

and, therefore, it causes more frequent action potentials. Parasympathetic stimulation has the opposite effect.

A chronotropic agent is one that increases (positive chronotrope) or decreases (negative chronotrope) the heart rate (Fig. 2.30). An inotropic agent is one that increases (positive inotrope) or decreases (negative inotrope) the force of contraction (contractility). The action potential varies in different myocytes. Fig. 2.31 shows the action potentials through the conduction pathway.

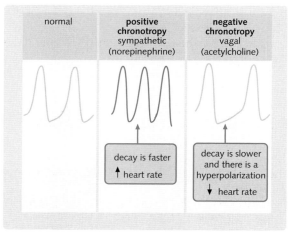

Fig. 2.30 Positive and negative chronotropy. Chronotropes affect the rate at which the heart beats.

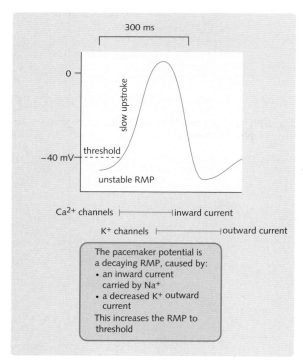

Fig. 2.29 The sinoatrial (SA) node action potential and the generation of the natural pacemaker potential. Voltage-gated calcium channels open once the resting membrane potential (RMP) has reached threshold.

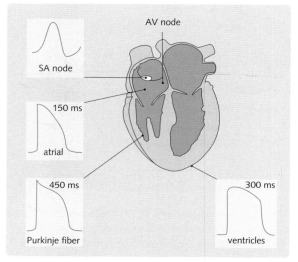

Fig. 2.31 Action potentials in different cardiac myocytes (SA, sinoatrial).

Excitation–contraction coupling

Contraction of cardiac muscle occurs in a similar manner to that of skeletal muscle.

Myosin projects from the thick filaments, and, when activated by Ca^{2+} and adenosine triphosphate (ATP), they pull the thin filaments (actin) together to cause sarcomere shortening. This process involves troponin C and tropomyosin. Full details of this can be found in *Crash Course: Musculoskeletal System*.

Contraction is initiated by a rise in cytoplasmic Ca^{2+}, because the contractile proteins are dependent upon Ca^{2+} (Fig. 2.32). Relaxation is brought about by a decrease in intracellular Ca^{2+} concentration (written $[Ca^{2+}]$) (Fig. 2.33), and so the duration of contraction is determined by the duration of the plateau. The force of contraction is directly related to $[Ca^{2+}]$ and contractile protein sensitivity to Ca^{2+}. The sensitivity is increased by the initial stretch of the sarcomere (Fig. 2.34).

Hence, the tension/Ca^{2+} curve is displaced to the left by an increased initial sarcomere length (i.e., tension produced during contraction is larger if the fibers are stretched initially; see Fig. 2.34). This is the basis for Starling's law of the heart.

Contraction is also dependent on ATP, which is supplied by the mitochondria.

Effect of inotropic agents

Inotropic agents increase force of contractility by affecting cytoplasmic (intracellular) Ca^{2+}. They increase cytoplasmic Ca^{2+} by:

- Increasing Ca^{2+} influx—norepinephrine increases Ca^{2+} entry by opening more Ca^{2+} channels.
- Decreasing Ca^{2+} removal—digitalis inhibits Na^+/K^+ ATPase and, therefore, reduces the Na^+ gradient. This, in turn, reduces the action of the Na^+–Ca^{2+} exchanger. This decreases Ca^{2+} removal from the cell.

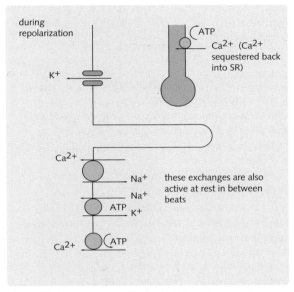

Fig. 2.33 Ion exchanges that take place during relaxation (SR, sarcoplasmic reticulum).

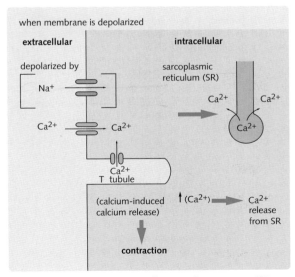

Fig. 2.32 Excitation and its effect on the myocyte (SR, sarcoplasmic reticulum).

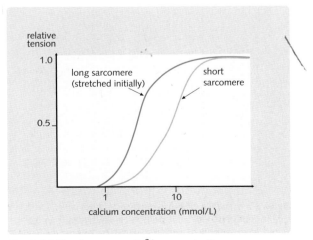

Fig. 2.34 Tension versus Ca^{2+} concentration.

Increased heart rate lessens the resting time that the cell has between beats. This decreases the amount of time available for Ca^{2+} removal, causing a gradual increase in cytoplasmic Ca^{2+} and, therefore, force. This is called the staircase or treppe effect (Fig. 2.35).

The cardiac cycle

Definition
The cardiac cycle (Fig. 2.36) is the sequence of pressure and volume changes that takes place during cardiac activity (Figs. 2.37–2.40). One cardiac cycle lasts about 0.9 seconds at rest.

Events of the cardiac cycle
Ventricular filling (diastole)
The atria and ventricles are all relaxed initially, and there is passive filling of the ventricles, driven by venous pressure. This causes ventricular volume, and therefore ventricular pressure, to rise. Contraction of the atria further increases the filling of the ventricles. However, this accounts for only about 15–20% of ventricular filling at rest. The volume now in the ventricle is termed the "end-diastolic volume."

Isovolumetric contraction (systole)
The contraction of the ventricles increases ventricular pressure. Once ventricular pressure rises

above atrial pressure, the atrioventricular valves close. This creates a closed chamber. As ventricular contraction proceeds, wall tension increases, causing a rapid rise in ventricular pressure. The rate of rise of pressure is a measure of cardiac contractility.

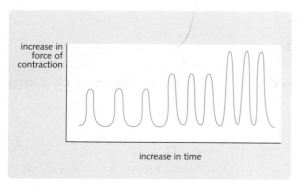

Fig. 2.35 Staircase or treppe effect. A gradual accumulation of Ca^{2+} within the myocytes leads to an increasing strength of contraction as the heart rate increases.

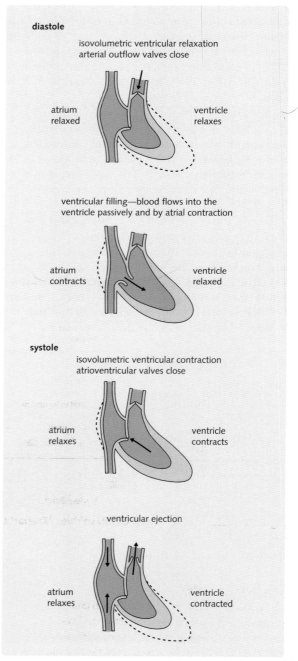

Fig. 2.36 The cardiac cycle.

The Cardiac cycle				
	Diastole	**Systole**		**Diastole**
Stage	Ventricular filling	Isovolumetric contraction	Election	Isovolumetric relaxation
Duration (s)	D.5	0.05	D.3	0.03
AV valves	Open	Closed	Closed	Closed
Arterial valves	Closed	Closed	Open	Closed
Ventricular pressure	Falls then slowly rises	Rapid rise	Rises then slowly falls	Rapid fall
Ventricular volume	Increases	Constant	Decreases	Constant

Fig. 2.37 Summary table of the stages of the cardiac cycle. Changes at fixed volume are referred to as isovolumetric, and precede the later contraction or dilation of the ventricles (AV, atrioventricular).

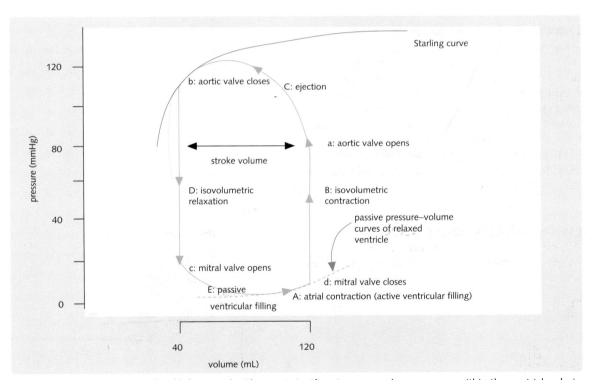

Fig. 2.38 Pressure–volume cycle of left ventricle. The most significant pressure changes occur within the ventricles during the isovolumetric stages.

Ejection (systole)

Ventricular pressure rises above arterial pressure, opening the arterial valves. This causes a rapid initial rise in arterial pressure, and then the pressure starts to fall as contraction fades.

The momentum of blood prevents immediate valve closure, even when ventricular pressure falls below arterial pressure. Eventually, the arterial valves close, which creates the brief rise in arterial pressure that is seen on the aortic pressure trace as a dicrotic notch.

23

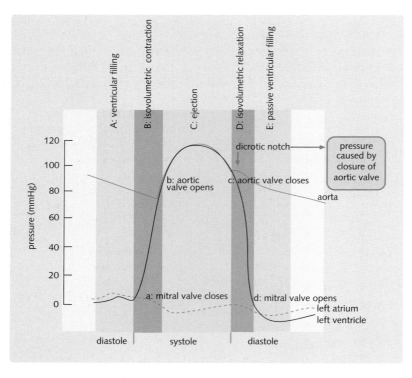

Fig. 2.39 Pressure and outflow in left side of heart. A. Pressure in the left ventricle increases slightly during left atrial contraction. B. The most rapid increase in pressure occurs during isovolumetric contraction. The increase in pressure caused by ventricular contraction closes the mitral valve (a). C. When left ventricular pressure just exceeds aortic pressure, the aortic valve opens (b) leading to ejection. Pressure rises to a peak and then falls, leading to aortic valve closure (c). D. Isovolumetric relaxation then occurs, and eventually left ventricular pressure is just below left atrial pressure, leading to the opening of the mitral valve (d). E. This allows passive filling of the ventricles.

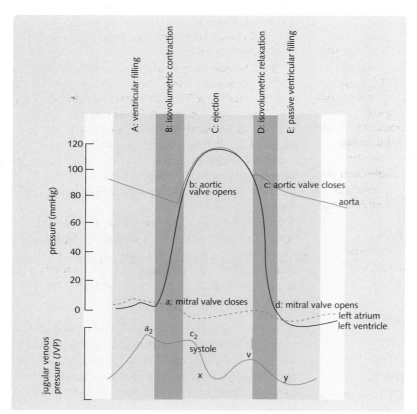

Fig. 2.40 Jugular venous pressure (JVP) and the cardiac cycle. The JVP reflects right atrial pressure due to the close proximity of the central veins to the right atrium and its activity (a_2, atrial contraction; c_2, movement of the tricuspid valve ring into the atrium when the ventricle contracts—in the jugular vein this may also be due to movement of the carotid artery in systole; v, peak pressure in the atrium due to atrial filling—the tricuspid valve is just about to open; x, x descent due to atrial relaxation; y, y descent due to ventricular filling).

The ventricle does not empty completely. In a normal heart, only about 50% of diastolic volume is ejected (ejection fraction [EF]). This remaining volume can be used to increase stroke volume when necessary; it can also be used as an indicator of ventricular performance.

Isovolumetric relaxation (diastole)

The closure of both sets of valves creates an enclosed chamber. The relaxation of sarcomeres plus collagen recoil drops the ventricular pressure. When ventricular pressure falls below atrial pressure, the atrioventricular valves open, leading to filling.

Cardiac cycle and normal heart sounds

Four heart sounds can be differentiated (Fig. 2.41):
- S_1—due to mitral and tricuspid valve closure (the atrioventricular valves).
- S_2—due to aortic and pulmonary valve closure (the semilunar/arterial valves).
- S_3—due to the sudden rapid flow of blood into the ventricles in diastole.
- S_4—due to flow of blood into the ventricles due to atrial systole (contraction).

Usually, only the first and second heart sounds are audible as a "lubb–dupp" every beat.

The second heart sound can be split (A_2:P_2), appearing to be two different distinguishable sounds. This is caused by inspiration increasing right ventricular filling and, therefore, increasing the time taken for right ventricular ejection and delaying pulmonary valve closure (P_2). Left ventricular ejection time is shortened, leading to faster closure of the aortic valve (A_2). This is termed "physiologic splitting." It is normal but may be altered in certain disease states.

Valvular abnormalities (stenosis and incompetence) lead to murmurs, with turbulent blood flow causing extra sounds. See Chapter 7, p. 144 for further discussion.

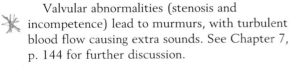

Electrical properties of the heart

Conduction system

The conduction system (Figs. 2.42 and 2.43) allows atrial and ventricular contraction to be coordinated for maximum efficiency.

The sequence of depolarization of the heart is as follows:
1. Depolarization is initiated in the SA node.
2. Depolarization spreads through adjacent atrial muscle cells, causing atrial systole in both atria.
3. At the AV node (the beginning of the only electrical pathway through the fibrotendinous ring), the wave of depolarization is delayed by approximately 0.1 second, so that the atria can contract fully.
4. Conduction continues through the bundle of His and its left and right bundle branches. These are very fast conduction pathways.
5. Numerous subendocardial Purkinje fibers distribute the impulse to the muscle cells in the endocardium.
6. Adjacent muscle cells then continue the spread to the epicardium to depolarize the whole ventricle.

All cells involved in the conduction process are muscle cells (not nerves), but not all (Purkinje cells, nodal cells) are contractile. They act as an electrical syncytium, because they have low-resistance electrical connections between them (gap junctions in the intercalated disc).

The SA node controls the heart rate because it has the fastest intrinsic firing rate, but the cells of the AV node and bundle of His can depolarize spontaneously at a slower rate and become pacemakers if the SA node ceases to function. Sometimes this occurs in cases of heart block, where the impulse is not conducted properly through the fibrotendinous ring. Ventricular contraction then occurs at a rate (about 40 beats/min) independent of atrial contraction.

Heart block is said to occur if there is slow or absent conduction in an area of the myocardium, usually in or around the AV node. In this case, the action potential can take longer to reach an area of the myocardium, and rhythm disturbances can result. These are called arrhythmias.

Re-entry occurs when the wave of depolarization travels back to re-excite an area of muscle that has already been depolarized and has recovered (Fig. 2.44). This usually happens as a consequence of ischemic damage to an area of myocardium. Again, this results in an arrhythmia.

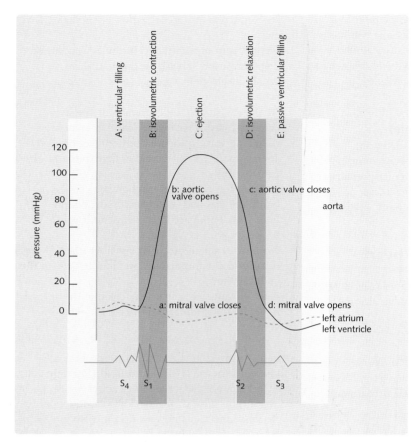

Fig. 2.41 The cardiac cycle and the heart sounds (S_1, closure of the mitral and tricuspid valves "lubb"; S_2, closure of the aortic and pulmonary valves "dupp"; S_3, passive ventricular filling—a low-frequency sound; S_4, active ventricular filling due to atrial contraction—a low-frequency sound).

Electrocardiography

The electrical activity of the heart can be measured by performing an electrocardiogram (ECG). This uses electrodes placed on the skin to detect the changing electrical potential within the tissue of the heart.

The characteristic elements of an ECG are:

- P wave—due to atrial depolarization and contraction.
- PR interval—measured from the beginning of the P wave to the beginning of the QRS complex; it is due to conduction through the AV node (approximately 120 msec).
- QRS complex—due to ventricular depolarization and repolarization (approximately 80 msec).
- QT interval—measured from the beginning of the QRS complex to the end of the T wave. It is due to ventricular muscle depolarization (approximately 300 ms).

Fiber size diameter conduction velocity		
Muscle cell (myocyte)	Diameter (mm)	Conduction velocity (m/s)
Atrial myocyte	10	1
AV node	3	0.05
Purkinje fibers	75	5
Ventricular myocyte	10–20	1

Fig. 2.42 Fiber diameter and conduction velocity of the different cardiac cells.

- T wave—due to ventricular repolarization.

These can be related to the cardiac cycle (Fig. 2.45), and their significance is explained fully in Chapter 8 on p. 150.

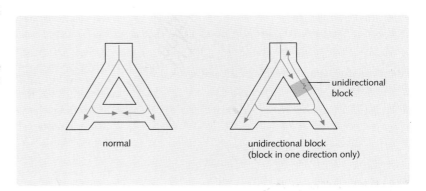

Fig. 2.43 Cardiac conduction pathway. The action potential is initiated in the sinoatrial (SA) node and spreads throughout both atria. It travels through the atrioventricular (AV) node, where it is delayed, and then to the bundle of His. From here, it travels down the left and right bundle branches and into Purkinje fibers. The action potential is then spread throughout the ventricles.

Fig. 2.44 Diagram illustrating heart block and re-entry. The direction of the impulse is indicated by the arrow. A block results from slow or absent conduction. Re-entry results from re-excitation of a region of the heart that has already contracted in the cardiac cycle. It depends upon the presence of a unidirectional block, and it is related to slow conduction and a short refractory period (redrawn from *Integrated Pharmacology* by Page CP, Curtis MJ, Sutter MC, et al. [eds], St. Louis, Mosby, 1997).

Control of cardiac output

Definitions and concepts

Definitions include:
- Cardiac output (CO)—the volume of blood ejected by one ventricle in 1 minute.
- Stroke volume (SV)—the volume of blood ejected in one ventricular contraction.
- Stroke work (SW)—the amount of external energy expended in one ventricular contraction. SW is the arterial pressure (AP) multiplied by the SV.

Total mechanical work equals the area within the pressure–volume loop (see Fig. 2.38). To calculate total energy expended, you must add internal work

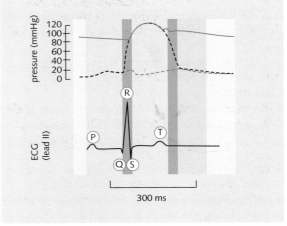

Fig. 2.45 ECG and the cardiac cycle (see Figs. 2.37 and 2.39 for the stages of the cardiac cycle).

(i.e., work during isovolumetric contraction), external work (i.e., SW), and heat.

Other definitions are:

- Contractility—the force of contraction for a given fiber length.
- Heart rate (HR)—the number of ventricular contractions in 1 minute.
- End-diastolic volume (EDV)—the volume of blood in the ventricle just before contraction.
- End-diastolic pressure (EDP)—the pressure of blood in the ventricle just before contraction (also called preload—see information to follow).
- End-systolic volume (ESV)—the volume of blood left in the ventricle after ejection.
- Central venous pressure (CVP)—the pressure of blood in the great veins as they enter the right atrium.
- Venous return (VR) —the volume of blood returning to the right heart in 1 minute.
- Total peripheral resistance (TPR)—the resistance to the flow of blood in the whole system. It is AP divided by the CO.
- Ejection fraction—the proportion of EDV that is ejected by contraction ([ESV/EDV] × 100).

The main equations governing CO and work are:

$$CO = SV \times HR$$

$$TPR = \frac{AP}{CO}$$

$$SW = SV \times AP$$

Only three things directly affect CO:

- End-diastolic volume of the right heart (i.e., preload, initial fiber length; this does not apply in pulmonary artery obstruction).
- Resistance to outflow.
- Functional state of the heart–lung unit.

Because CO is a product of SV and HR, changes in SV will affect CO. SV is governed by:

- Initial stretch—see Starling's law of the heart (right column).
- Contractility.
- AP, which opposes ejection of blood.

Remember that cardiac output is limited by venous return—without integrated regulation of the cardiovascular system, an increased heart rate will be compensated by reduced stroke volume due to inadequate ventricular filling. This also applies in shock.

Starling's law of the heart

"The energy released during contraction depends upon the initial fiber length" (Fig. 2.46). The greater the heart is stretched by filling, then the greater the energy released by contraction. This phenomenon is due to the stretch-dependent sensitivity of myocardial contractile proteins to Ca^{2+}, and it is known as Starling's law of the heart (Starling's law).

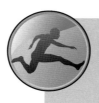 Think of the heart muscle as an elastic band—the more you stretch it initially, the farther you can fire it. This will help you understand Starling's law.

Although the initial stretch of the myocardium is produced by the EDV, EDP is easier to measure, and the relationship between the two is almost linear. EDP plotted against SV produces the Starling curve (Fig. 2.47). Excessively high filling pressures will cause excessive distension, and the relationship is no longer valid. EDP in the right ventricle is closely related to CVP.

Starling's law matches right and left ventricular stroke volumes. If HR and myocardial contractility are constant, CVP will determine CO. Although CVP affects the right ventricle, within a few beats the venous pressure will change in the pulmonary circulation, and so the filling pressure of the left ventricle will also be affected, and left ventricular output will change according to the stretch produced by the new EDV. Remember that the circulatory system is closed, with the two ventricles in series. Cardiac output must equal venous return, and discrepancies between left and right ventricular output can only be transient in the steady state. Pathologic changes may produce inequalities, such as left-sided (or congestive) heart failure producing pulmonary edema.

Preload and afterload are important factors affecting stroke volume, and hence CO. Although the ideas originate from isolated muscle experiments, they have been applied to the study of the heart *in vivo*:

- Preload is the force associated with the degree of initial stretch in the ventricle due to the initial volume load. It is determined by the EDV, which

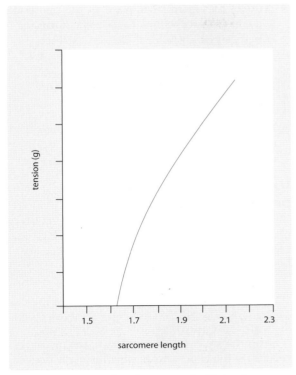

Fig. 2.46 Sarcomere length compared with tension. Increasing the initial sarcomere length increases tension, up to the maximum stretch possible for an individual myocyte.

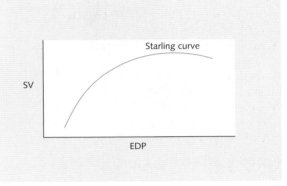

Fig. 2.47 Stroke volume (SV) compared with end-diastolic pressure (EDP). This produces the Starling curve, which shows that an increase in EDP (and therefore end-diastolic volume [EDV] as they have an almost linear relationship) causes an increased SV. There is, however, a limit at which the curve turns downward and the relationship is no longer valid. The mechanism for this downturn is complex, and it mainly reflects excessive dilatation of the ventricle and valvular regurgitation.

is related to EDP. In the right side of the heart, EDP is almost equal to CVP.

- Afterload is the force (load in systole) that is determined by AP (which is related to the resistance to outflow [i.e., TPR]) and ventricular volume by the Laplace relationship.

An increase in preload will increase CO according to Starling's law. An increase in afterload will initially decrease CO. The heart will have a greater residual volume after contraction. If the filling pressure remains constant, the greater residual volume will distend the ventricle further, and the next contraction will be stronger. This is an attempt to restore the CO.

Starling's experiments were conducted on an isolated heart–lung preparation in 1914 (Fig. 2.48). Although it is not possible to monitor the determinants of CO in the way Starling could by isolating the heart and lungs,

cardiologists can insert a single catheter from the femoral artery up the aorta and into the left ventricle by passing it retrogradely through the aortic valve. The catheter contains conductance sensors to measure left ventricular volume and a pressure sensor at the tip. This records the pressure–volume loops (Fig. 2.49).

Starling's findings in the controlled situation of the isolated heart–lung preparation are important in enabling clinicians to understand the significance of:

- Adequate, but not excessive, filling of the ventricles (e.g., in heart failure, high EDV may be pathologic).
- Keeping peripheral resistance as low as possible to maximize CO.
- Maintaining a sufficient level of contractility to maintain life when the previous determinants have been optimized.

When the blood supply through the coronary arteries is compromised, it is important to keep certain methods of increasing CO (especially increased contractility) to a minimum, because they increase oxygen consumption of the heart muscle. This increased oxygen demand cannot be met by an increase in myocardial blood flow and thus results in ischemia.

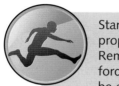

Starling's law reflects the innate properties of the myocytes. Remember, however, that the force of contraction can also be affected by extrinsic factors (e.g., sympathetic stimulation). Starling's law is not the only factor that affects SV.

Factors affecting contractility

Numerous factors can affect the myocyte and alter contractility (Fig. 2.50). The force of contraction is affected by other variables in addition to that of initial fiber length (Starling mechanism; Fig. 2.51). The term inotropic is also used to denote the contractility of the heart. Positive inotropes (increased contractility) include:

- Sympathetic stimulation. Norepinephrine from sympathetic nerves binds to β_1-receptors on cardiac myocytes and increases intracellular Ca^{2+} by cyclic adenosine monophosphate (cAMP)-activated protein kinase A and G-protein linked Ca^{2+} channels. This increases the force of contraction and slightly shortens systole.

- Plasma Ca^{2+}. Increases in plasma Ca^{2+} can result in increased sarcoplasmic Ca^{2+} in the myocytes.
- Drugs: cardiac glycosides—digoxin, ouabain; β_1-agonists—epinephrine, isoproterenol, dobutamine; and some antiarrhythmics.

Negative inotropes include:
- Disease (e.g., ischemia, hypoxia).
- Acidity.
- Drugs: β_1-blockers (e.g., propranolol, atenolol), Ca^{2+}-channel blockers (e.g., verapamil), barbiturates, and most general anesthetic agents.

Venous return, central venous pressure, and cardiac output

Venous return (VR) depends on the mean circulatory filling pressure (P_{mc}), right atrial pressure (P_{ra}), and venous resistance (R_v), according to the following formula:

$$VR = \frac{(P_{mc} - P_{ra})}{R_v}$$

Right atrial pressure is equivalent to the central venous pressure in the normal heart. The mean circulatory filling pressure is experimentally derived, and it is the pressure that would result throughout the circulatory system if the heart were to stop

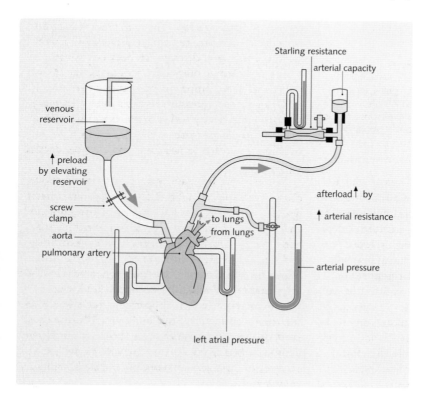

Fig. 2.48 Starling heart–lung preparation. Using an isolated heart–lung preparation, Starling examined the effects of varying end-diastolic volumes (EDV) and arterial resistance in stroke volume. In practicality, EDV is an index of preload, and arterial resistance is an index of afterload. These terms were not used by Starling in his experiments, but they are sometimes used now. (Redrawn with permission of the Physiological Society.)

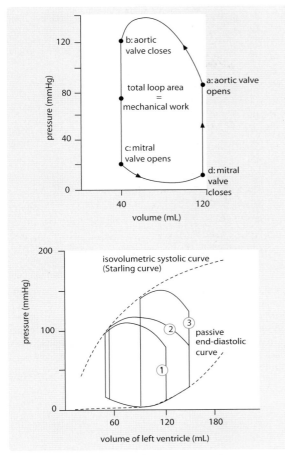

Fig. 2.49 Pressure–volume loops (1, normal state; 2, increased end-diastolic volume [EDV] leads to increased stroke volume [SV] if arterial pressure is constant; 3, increased EDV and increased AP result in a decreased SV). The end-systolic points of the loops produce the Starling curve so long as the contractility remains constant.

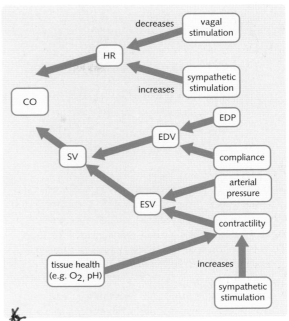

Fig. 2.50 Summary of the factors affecting cardiac output (CO, cardiac output; EDP, end-diastolic pressure; EDV, end-diastolic volume; HR, heart rate; ESV, end-systolic volume; SV, stroke volume).

beating. It is determined principally by the blood volume and the degree of sympathetic activation (Fig. 2.52). The effect of sympathetic activation is to decrease the total cross-sectional area of the circulatory system. This should not be confused with TPR, which is a separate and distinct variable.

The equation is the equivalent of the previous description of arterial blood flow (i.e., flow [venous return] is equal to the pressure gradient between the central veins and the systemic circulation divided by the resistance). In a normal, healthy individual, any changes are automatically compensated for. For example, an increased right atrial pressure leads to reduced venous return, but it also leads to increased

output by Starling's law. This will then reduce the right atrial pressure, restoring equilibrium. There may be a transient discrepancy between venous return and cardiac output (as strictly defined), but remember that compensation occurs automatically. If the right atrial pressure remains raised, increased sympathetic activity will increase the mean filling pressure to compensate, producing a new equilibrium with a higher CVP and a higher cardiac output.

The effects of disease and resulting compensatory changes are shown in Fig. 2.53. In right-sided heart disease, where myocardial function is compromised and right atrial pressure is persistently raised, the body compensates by increasing sympathetic drive and retaining fluid to increase blood volume (Fig. 2.53, A). Common treatments for this situation are diuretics and vasodilators, which relax the system, as indicated in Fig. 2.53, B, and help remove the excess fluid. In hypovolemic shock, a reduction in blood volume is also associated with sympathetic activation (Fig. 2.53, C, D). The effects of the changes in hypovolemic shock on cardiac function are shown in Fig. 2.54.

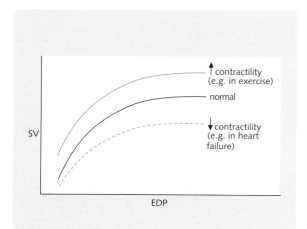

Fig. 2.51 Contractility and the Starling curve. Changes in contractility are characterized by upward (positively inotropic) and downward (negatively inotropic) displacement of the Starling curve (EDP, end-diastolic pressure; SV, stroke volume).

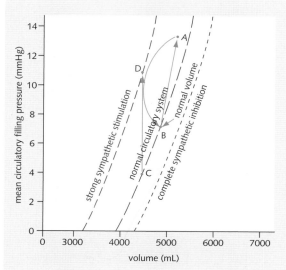

Fig. 2.53 A. Examples of compensatory changes in mean circulatory filling pressure in disease. Compensatory changes in chronic heart disease, where volume increases and sympathetic stimulation increases mean filling pressure. B. Treatment is to counter these changes and unload the heart. C and D. In hemorrhagic shock, the blood loss is countered by sympathetic activation (see Fig. 2.54).

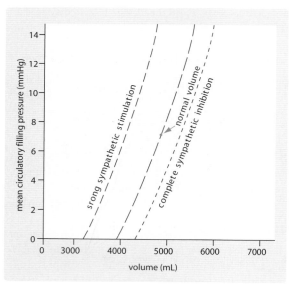

Fig. 2.52 The effects of volume and sympathetic activation on the mean circulatory filling pressure (P_{mc}). The mean filling pressure depends on the degree of filling (volume) and the stiffness of the compartment, often referred to as the tone. The reciprocal of the stiffness is called capacitance, compliance, or distensibility. The tone is increased by sympathetic stimulation, which shifts the curve to the left (vasoconstriction/venoconstriction) so that there is a higher filling pressure for a given volume (redrawn with permission from *Textbook of Medical Physiology*, 9th ed. by Guyton AC, Hall JE, Philadelphia, W.B. Saunders, 1995).

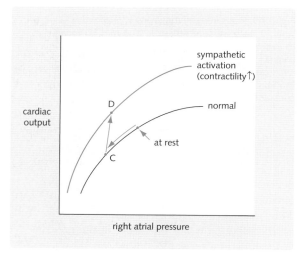

Fig. 2.54 Cardiac function curve showing the changes in hemorrhagic shock. Fluid loss causes a fall in cardiac filling (C), reducing right atrial pressure. Cardiac output will then fall, but increased sympathetic activity will increase contractility (moving the Starling curve upward and to the left) while also causing venoconstriction, which will increase venous return and hence raise right atrial pressure.

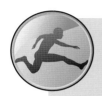

Venous return = right heart input and output = pulmonary blood flow = left heart input and output = systemic blood flow BECAUSE THEY ARE ALL **IN SERIES**.

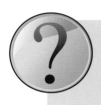

- Describe the anatomy of the heart, especially the following:
    - (a). Gross structure of the atrium and ventricles, both internal and external.
    - (b). Relations of the heart to the other structures in the mediastinum.
    - (c). Blood supply and drainage.
    - (d). Great vessels.
- Describe the embryology of the following:
    - (a). The fusion of the heart tubes and subsequent development into the four chambers.
    - (b). The formation of the interatrial and interventricular septa, including the congenital defects that may arise.
    - (c). How the outflow tracts develop.
- Identify the tissue layers of the heart.
- Describe the heart skeleton and its function.
- Describe the structure of a typical valve.
- List the different types of cardiac myocytes, and explain the ways in which they differ.
- Draw a basic diagram of a cardiac muscle cell and the arrangement with neighboring cells.
- Sketch the internal structure of a cardiac muscle cell, including myofibrils.
- Define the resting membrane potential and the factors that influence it.
- Sketch the action potential produced in the different cells of the myocardium, and explain the contribution of the different ion channels.
- Explain the pacemaker potential and how it is generated.
- Explain the role of Ca^{2+} in excitation–contraction coupling.
- Identify the phases of the cardiac cycle.
- Explain the pressure changes during these cycles. Sketch the ventricular pressure–volume loop.
- Describe how jugular venous pressure changes with the events of the cardiac cycle.
- Sketch the conduction pathway.
- Define the terms cardiac output (CO), stroke volume (SV), stroke work (SW), heart rate (HR), end-diastolic volume (EDV), end-diastolic pressure (EDP), endo-systolic pressure (ESP), central venous pressure (CVP), venous return (VR), total peripheral resistance (TPR), and contractility.
- State Starling's law of the heart. Explain its physiologic significance.
- Draw a ventricular function curve, and show how it can be changed by disease.
- Give an example of an inotropic agent, and describe the physiological factors that affect contractility.

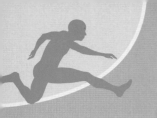

3. Structure and Function of the Vessels

Organization of the vessels

Classification of the vessels

The circulatory system is composed of vessels designed for:

- Conductance.
- Resistance.
- Exchange.
- Capacitance.

Conductance

These are low-resistance vessels, which are large arteries with predominantly elastic walls. Their role is delivery of blood to more distal vessels, although they also have a small resistance role.

Resistance

These vessels are the terminal arteries and arterioles, and they are the main resistance to blood flow.

Resistance vessels act to control local blood flow and maintain arterial pressure. Dilatation of these vessels lowers resistance and increases blood flow (vasodilatation). Constriction of these vessels increases resistance and decreases blood flow (vasoconstriction). They can, therefore, influence the exchange vessels by governing the flow that reaches them.

Exchange

These vessels are the numerous capillaries that have very thin walls. This optimizes their function, which is to allow rapid transfer between blood and tissues.

Capacitance

These vessels are thin-walled, low-resistance venules and veins. They act as a variable reservoir of blood and contain almost two thirds of the blood volume in a normal individual at rest. These veins are innervated by venoconstrictor fibers which, when stimulated, can displace the blood into the heart.

Vasculature

The vasculature (Fig. 3.1) can be classified anatomically into:

- Elastic arteries (e.g., aorta and common carotids).
- Muscular arteries (e.g., coronary, cerebral, and popliteal arteries).
- Arterioles.
- Capillaries.
- Postcapillary venules.
- Muscular venules.
- Veins.

The main function of the arteries and arterioles is to deliver blood to the capillaries. In the capillaries, exchange with and filtration into the interstitial fluid take place. Fluid and metabolites return to the heart

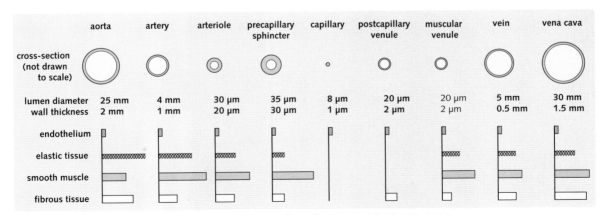

Fig. 3.1 Vessels of the circulation (adapted from *Physiol Rev* by Burton AC 34:619, 1954).

through veins and lymphatic vessels. Veins return blood to the heart, and the lymphatic system returns excess filtrate to the blood.

Anatomy of the circulatory system

The anatomy of the circulatory system is shown in Figs. 3.2–3.14.

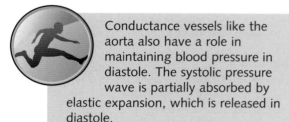

Conductance vessels like the aorta also have a role in maintaining blood pressure in diastole. The systolic pressure wave is partially absorbed by elastic expansion, which is released in diastole.

Development of the circulation

The vasculature develops from the angioblastic cords of mesoderm. The aortic ends of the primitive heart tube become the aortic arches and dorsal aortae. The aortic arches develop into the great arteries of the neck and thorax, whereas the dorsal aortae produce the following branches:

- Ventral branches (derived from the remnants of the vitelline arteries). These supply the gastrointestinal tract.
- Lateral branches. These supply retroperitoneal structures (e.g., kidneys).
- Intersegmental branches. These supply the rest of the body.

The paired dorsal aortae connect to the umbilical arteries, which carry blood to the placenta.

Text continued on p. 42

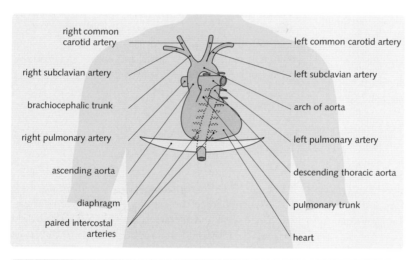

Fig. 3.2 Arteries of the thorax.

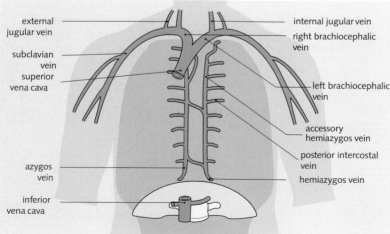

Fig. 3.3 Veins of the thorax.

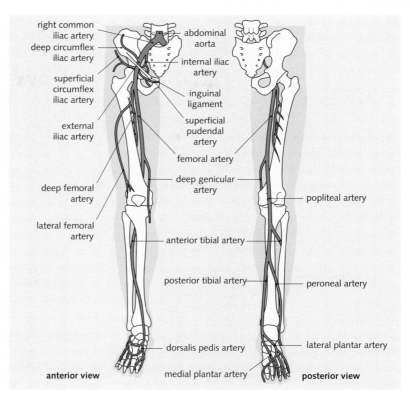

Fig. 3.13 Arteries of the lower limbs.

In the figure above, the following labels appear:

right common iliac artery
deep circumflex iliac artery
superficial circumflex iliac artery
external iliac artery
deep femoral artery
lateral femoral artery
abdominal aorta
internal iliac artery
inguinal ligament
superficial pudendal artery
femoral artery
deep genicular artery
popliteal artery
anterior tibial artery
posterior tibial artery
peroneal artery
dorsalis pedis artery
lateral plantar artery
medial plantar artery
anterior view
posterior view

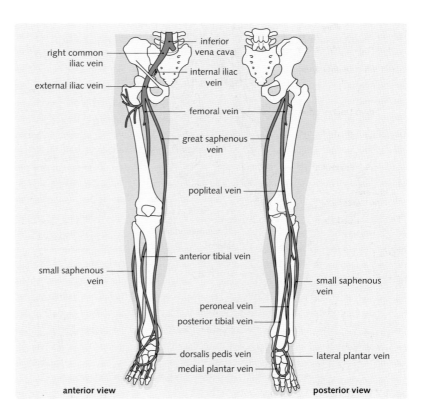

Fig. 3.14 Veins of the lower limbs.

In the figure above, the following labels appear:

right common iliac vein
external iliac vein
inferior vena cava
internal iliac vein
femoral vein
great saphenous vein
popliteal vein
anterior tibial vein
small saphenous vein
small saphenous vein
peroneal vein
posterior tibial vein
dorsalis pedis vein
medial plantar vein
lateral plantar vein
anterior view
posterior view

41

The venous system consists of three components, which are initially paired:

- Cardinal system. This drains the head, neck, body wall, and limbs.
- Vitelline veins. These drain the yolk sac.
- Umbilical veins. These carry blood from the placenta to the embryo.

Initially, the venous system drains into the sinus horns, but eventually it drains into the venae cavae and right atrium. In general, it is the right-sided veins that persist while the left-sided veins regress during gestation, and so systemic venous drainage is via the vena cava to the right side of the heart. However, it is the left umbilical vein that persists while the right umbilical vein disappears.

In the liver, the vitelline system forms the ductus venosus, which shunts blood from the umbilical vein directly into the inferior vena cava during gestation. This is vital, because it allows oxygenated blood to enter the right atrium of the heart, pass predominantly through the foramen ovale, and then be pumped around the fetus (Fig. 3.15).

The foramen ovale enables the oxygenated blood in the right atrium to pass into the left atrium and reach the systemic circulation.

The ductus arteriosus develops from the sixth aortic arch. It connects the pulmonary arteries to the descending aorta. This allows oxygenated blood pumped into the pulmonary arteries to enter the systemic circulation. (Because the lungs are not functional during gestation, there is no need for a large pulmonary circulation.) The ductus is kept open during fetal life by circulating prostaglandins.

The head receives a preferential blood supply. Therefore, if there is a decrease in umbilical artery supply, the head will continue to receive an adequate blood supply at the expense of the rest of the body (i.e., the head grows but the body does not).

Deoxygenated blood returns to the placenta through the umbilical arteries, which connect to the aorta.

Circulatory adaptations at birth

A series of changes convert the single system of blood flow around the fetus into dual systems at birth.

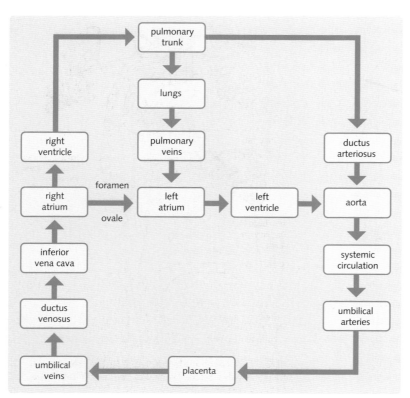

Fig. 3.15 Fetal blood pathway.

Blood flow in the umbilical vessels drastically declines in the 3–4 minutes after birth because of:
- Compression of the cord.
- Vasoconstriction in response to cold, mechanical stimuli, and/or catecholamines.

At birth, the pulmonary vascular resistance falls rapidly because:
- The mechanical effect of ventilation opens the constricted alveolar vessels.
- Raising PO_2 and lowering PCO_2 causes vasodilatation of the pulmonary vessels.

This produces an increase in the pulmonary blood flow.

The sudden cessation of umbilical blood flow and the opening of the pulmonary system cause a change in the pressure balance in the atria. There is a pressure drop in the right atrium and a pressure rise in the left atrium (caused by an increased pulmonary venous return to the left atrium and elevated systemic vascular resistance). This reverses the pressure gradient across the atria and forces the flexible septum primum against the rigid septum secundum, closing the foramen ovale. These two septa will normally fuse together after about 3 months.

The ductus venosus closes soon after birth (Figs. 3.16 and 3.17). The mechanism is unclear, but it may involve prostaglandin inhibition.

The closure is not vital to life because the umbilical vein no longer carries any blood.

The ductus arteriosus closes 1–8 days after birth. It is thought that as the pulmonary circulation fills, the pressure drop in the pulmonary trunk causes blood to flow from the aorta into the pulmonary trunk through the ductus arteriosus. This blood is oxygenated, and the increase in PO_2 causes the smooth muscle in the wall of the ductus to constrict. This obstructs flow in the ductus arteriosus.

Eventually, the intima of the ductus arteriosus thickens—complete obliteration of the ductus results in the formation of the ligamentum arteriosum, which attaches the pulmonary trunk to the aorta.

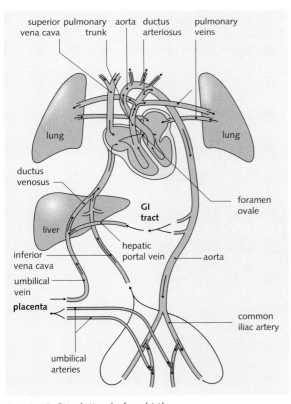

Fig. 3.16 Circulation before birth.

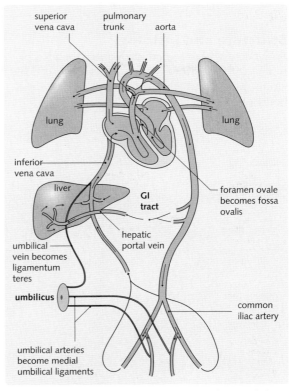

Fig. 3.17 Circulation after birth. Note the closure of the foramen ovale, ductus arteriosus, ductus venosus, and umbilical vessels closing off the fetal shunts.

Congenital vascular abnormalities

Many circulatory anomalies can develop, but few of these conditions cause any problems. Those that do include:

- Patent ductus arteriosus. This occurs when the ductus arteriosus fails to close.
- Coarctation of the aorta. This is abnormal stenotic thickening of the aorta that affects systemic blood flow.
- Persistent patent foramen ovale. This is caused by a failure of fusion of the septum primum and septum secundum, leading to a permanent shunt between the atria.

Further information about these anomalies can be found in Chapter 5, beginning on p. 108.

 The components of a vessel wall reflect that vessel's function. For example, if a vessel wall contains many elastic fibers, it will be better suited to act as a conductance vessel.

Structure and histology

A blood vessel has an endothelium surrounded by three main layers (or tunicae). These are called the intima, media, and adventitia. Fig. 3.18 shows the layers of a typical vessel.

Arteries and veins

An elastic artery consists of concentric layers of elastin and smooth muscle, whereas a muscular artery has prominent muscular media, with internal and external elastic laminae. In contrast, a vein has a thin media. Fig. 3.19 shows the structure of an elastic artery, a muscular artery, and a vein.

Capillary

The structure of a capillary is shown in Fig. 3.20.

Lymphatic vessel

The structure of a lymphatic capillary is shown in Fig. 3.21.

Vascular endothelium and smooth muscle

Functions of endothelial cells

Endothelial cells are involved in a number of processes, including:

- Transportation of substances between interstitium and plasma.
- Providing a low-friction surface for blood flow.
- Regulation of clotting.
- Inflammatory responses.
- Control of vascular tone.

Some of these functions require the secretion of a variety of substances (Fig. 3.22).

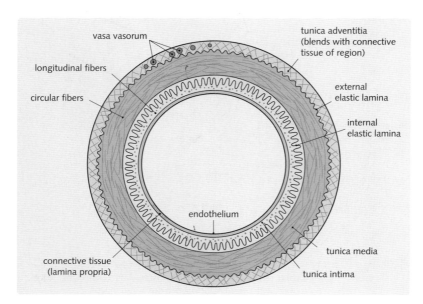

Fig. 3.18 Cross-section of a generic vessel showing the order of the layers.

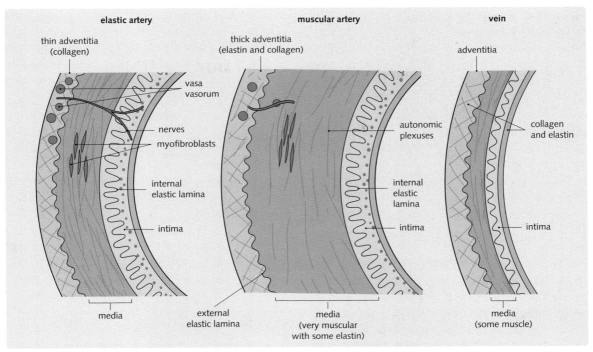

Fig. 3.19 Cross-sections of walls of elastic arteries, muscular arteries, and veins.

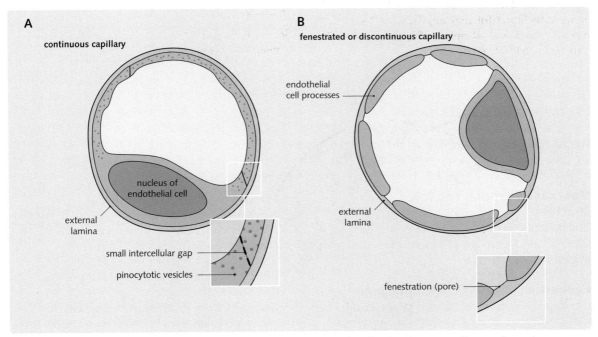

Fig. 3.20 Cross-sections of capillaries with continuous and fenestrated walls. Continuous capillary walls are less permeable than fenestrated capillary walls (redrawn from *Human Histology*, 2nd ed. by Stevens A, Lowe J, St. Louis, Mosby, 1997).

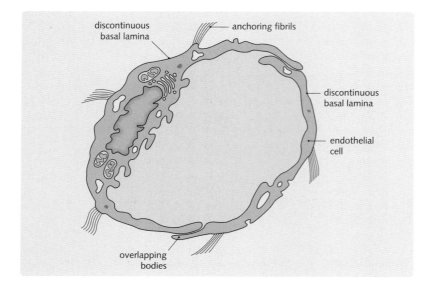

Fig. 3.21 Cross-section of a lymph capillary. Lymph capillaries are designed to allow flow only into the lumen. Overlapping endothelial cells operate as one-way valves to accomplish this. Anchoring filaments connect the endothelial cells to the surrounding tissue. When surrounding tissues are swollen with excess interstitial fluid (e.g., in inflammation), the filaments pull the endothelial cells apart to increase lymphatic flow. The discontinuous basal lamina (basement membrane) also allows greater movement of fluids and solutes.

Secreted factors and their functions	
Factor secreted	**Function**
Structural components	To form the basal lamina
Prostacyclin	Vasodilatation; inhibits platelet aggregation
Nitric oxide	Vasodilatation; inhibits adhesion and aggregation
Angiotensin-converting enzyme*	Converts angiotensin I to II; degrades bradykinin and serokinin
Platelet activating factor	Activates platelets and neutrophils
Tissue plasminogen activator (tPA)	Regulates fibrinolysis
Thromboplastin	Promotes coagulation
Von Willebrand's factor	Promotes platelet adhesion and clotting

*Actually located on the surface on endothelial cells.

Fig. 3.22 Some factors secreted from endothelial cells and their functions.

Vascular smooth muscle
Structure
The structure of smooth muscle is shown in Fig. 3.23. A mass of smooth muscle functions as if it were a single unit.

Contraction of vascular smooth muscle
Contraction is initiated by a rise in intracellular Ca^{2+}. This leads to an actin–myosin interaction, which causes shortening and tension. The process differs from that of the myocardium in the following ways:

- Myosin light chain phosphorylation. Unlike skeletal or cardiac muscle, the myosin in vascular smooth muscle only becomes active if its light chains are phosphorylated. The enzyme is activated by a calcium–calmodulin complex, which is dependent on a rise in intracellular Ca^{2+} for its formation.
- Sustained actin–myosin interactions enable vascular smooth muscle to maintain tension for much less energy than that needed by skeletal muscle. The actin–myosin interactions are long lasting because of slow myosin kinetics.

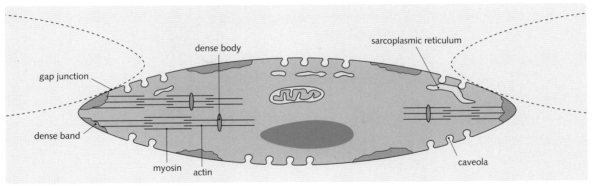

Fig. 3.23 Structure of smooth muscle cell. The actin–myosin filaments have been magnified (adapted from *Introducing Cardiovascular Physiology* by Levick R, New York, Butterworth–Heinemann, 1995).

- Sensitivity to intracellular Ca^{2+}. Chemical factors can alter the relationship between cytoplasmic Ca^{2+} and contractile force (i.e., the sensitivity of the contractile apparatus to Ca^{2+} can be changed). The cytoplasmic Ca^{2+} concentration and the resting membrane potential are dependent upon the state of ion-conducting channels (K^+, Ca^{2+}, and Cl^- channels).

Effect of sympathetic innervation

Fig. 3.24 shows the mechanism of sympathetic innervation.

Vascular smooth muscle relaxation

Vascular smooth muscle relaxation can be brought about by three (or possibly four) different mechanisms. Each mechanism relies upon reducing intracellular Ca^{2+}:

- Hyperpolarization. Hyperpolarizing the resting membrane reduces the number of open Ca^{2+} channels, leading to a decrease in intracellular Ca^{2+} concentration and relaxation. Hyperpolarization is caused by hypoxia, acidosis, calcitonin-gene-related peptide, and certain drugs (e.g., diazoxide, cromakalim, pinacidil).
- Cyclic adenosine monophosphate (cAMP)-mediated vasodilatation (Fig. 3.25).
- Cyclic guanosine monophosphate (cGMP)-mediated vasodilatation (Fig. 3.26).
- Sensitivity to intracellular Ca^{2+} is probably another cause of relaxation. This lowers the sensitivity of the contractile apparatus to the cytoplasmic Ca^{2+}, makes the contraction weaker for a given concentration of Ca^{2+}, and causes dilatation. Isoproterenol may work

in this way as well as with cAMP-mediated vasodilatation.

Hemodynamics in arteries and veins

Hemodynamics in arteries

In normal arteries and veins, there is laminar flow (Fig. 3.27). Turbulent flow occurs in the ventricles. Single-file flow occurs in capillaries. Although this is a simplistic view, it is sufficient for most basic purposes.

Norepinephrine contracts smooth muscle, whereas nitric oxide relaxes smooth muscle (NO, no contraction).

Pulse waveform

The difference between systolic and diastolic pressure is called the pulse pressure. The pressure wave created by ventricular ejection depends upon:

- Stroke volume.
- Heart rate.
- Elasticity of the arterial wall.
- Peripheral resistance.
- Blood volume.

The mean arterial pressure is the arterial pressure averaged over time. Mean arterial pressure is not just midway between diastolic and systolic pressure. The time spent in diastole is longer than that spent in

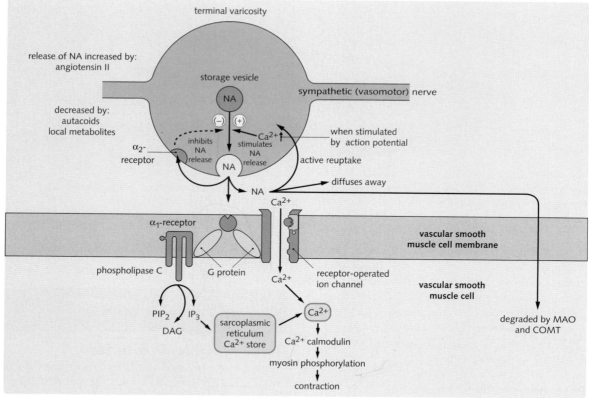

Fig. 3.24 Release of noradrenaline from a sympathetic junction and its effect on the vascular smooth muscle (VSM) cell. Sympathetic stimulation results in the release of noradrenaline from the sympathetic terminal varicosities. Noradrenaline acts on α_1-receptors on the VSM cells. This results in an increase in intracellular Ca^{2+} by directly opening Ca^{2+} channels and via a second messenger system releasing Ca^{2+} from the sarcoplasmic reticulum. It is the increase of intracellular Ca^{2+} that brings about contraction (AP, action potential; COMT, catechol O-methyltransferase; DAG, diacylglycerol; IP_3, inositol triphosphate; MAO, monoamine oxidase; PIP_2, phosphatidyl inositol bisphosphate).

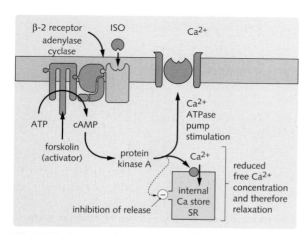

Fig. 3.25 cAMP-mediated vasodilatation as shown by the action of adrenaline (Ad) (ATP, adenosine triphosphate; SR, sarcoplasmic reticulum).

systole (Fig. 3.28). Thus, mean arterial pressure is closer to diastolic pressure. It is commonly approximated as one third of the pulse pressure added to diastolic pressure.

Measurement of arterial blood pressure

Arterial blood pressure can be directly measured by the use of invasive catheters. However, in most patients, blood pressure is determined indirectly by using a sphygmomanometer and the following procedure.

- Place the sphygmomanometer cuff around the patient's arm above the elbow. Ideally, do this while the patient is sitting or lying down.
- Palpate the radial or brachial artery and inflate the cuff until a pulse is no longer felt.
- Auscultate the brachial artery at the medial side of the antecubital fossa using a stethoscope. No sound should be heard at this point.

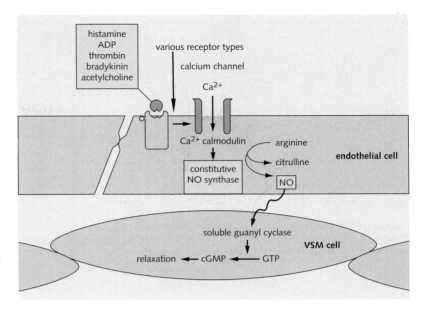

Fig. 3.26 cGMP-mediated vasodilatation as shown by the action of vasoactive mediators (ADP, adenosine diphosphate; GTP, guanosine triphosphate; NO, nitric oxide; VSM, vascular smooth muscle).

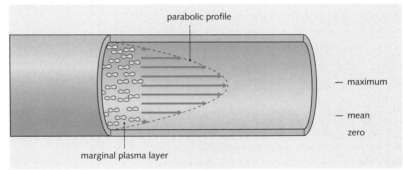

Fig. 3.27 The dynamics of laminar flow. Blood flows as if in sheets (laminae) with blood being faster in the middle than at the sides, where friction slows flow. The dashed line indicates the parabolic profile of the different speeds across the vessel. Cells tend to accumulate in the center of the flow, leaving a marginal plasma layer with fewer red cells at the periphery.

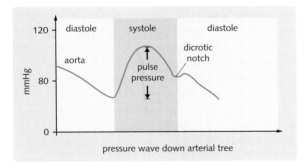

Fig. 3.28 Pulse waveform. The dicrotic notch is caused by closure of the aortic valve.

- Gradually lower the cuff pressure until a dull tapping sound is heard. The cuff pressure at this point represents systolic blood pressure.
- Continue lowering the cuff pressure until the tapping sound is no longer heard. The cuff pressure at the point where the sound disappears represents diastolic blood pressure.

Normal blood pressure

Normal blood pressure for a healthy adult male at rest is generally considered to be 120/80 mmHg. However, this value can vary because of many factors, and these must be taken into account when assessing a patient's blood pressure:

- Aging causes an increase in blood pressure because of decreased arterial compliance, often caused by arteriosclerosis. As a rough rule, systolic pressure should be no more than 100 mmHg plus age in years.
- During sleep, blood pressure falls, consistent with the body's decreased metabolic demands.
- Heavy dynamic exercise increases blood pressure because of increased cardiac output. However, the increase in blood pressure is less than 30% because of decreased total peripheral resistance.

49

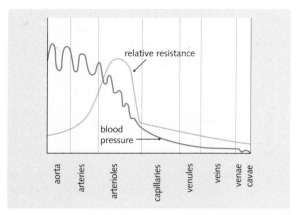

Fig. 3.29 How blood pressure and vascular resistance change across the vascular system. Pressure in the arterial side and in the great veins varies with the cardiac cycle.

- Heavy static exercise greatly increases blood pressure (possibly, by more than 30%) because of the exercise pressor response (described later).
- Anger, sexual excitement, and stress increase blood pressure, all because of sympathetically mediated responses.

Other factors that may cause changes in blood pressure include:

- Respiration. Mean arterial pressure may fall by a small amount during inspiration because of a transient fall in stroke volume (pulsus paradoxus).
- Pregnancy. Blood pressure normally falls gradually in the first trimester, reaching a minimum in the second trimester, and then rises to normal in the third trimester.
- Physiologic processes. For example, the Valsalva maneuver and the diving reflex.
- Pathologic processes. For example, shock, hemorrhage, and heart failure.

There is a physiologic fall in blood pressure from the major arteries through the vascular tree. Note that the largest pressure drop is at arteriolar level, the site of the main resistance to blood flow (Fig. 3.29).

Blood flow and velocity

Blood flow is defined as the volume of blood that flows through a given tissue in a given time. For the whole body, this must equal the cardiac output. Ohm's law states:

$$\text{Flow} = \frac{\text{(pressure difference)}}{\text{resistance (I = V/R)}}$$

Hence, the determinants of flow are the blood

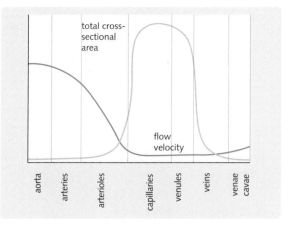

Fig. 3.30 Total cross-sectional area and velocity within the different anatomical classifications of vessels. Velocity in the arterial side actually varies with the cardiac cycle; the mean velocity is shown.

pressure across the length of a vessel (see previous discussion) and the resistance to flow within the vessel (see later discussion).

Velocity of blood flow

The velocity of blood flow is inversely related to the total cross-sectional area (Fig. 3.30). The branching nature of the circulatory system means that the total cross-sectional area of the capillaries is much greater than that of the arteries or veins. This reduces flow velocity in the capillaries.

Vascular resistance
Poiseuille's law

Poiseuille determined that resistance (R) to the flow of a fluid through a tube is proportional to the length of the tube (l), viscosity of the fluid (η), and inversely proportional to the radius of the tube to the fourth power (r^4). He stated:

$$R = \frac{8\eta l}{\pi r^4}$$

Using Ohm's law (I = V/R), we can derive:

$$\text{Flow} = \frac{\text{(pressure difference)} \times \pi r^4}{8\eta l}$$

From these equations, we can explain the resistance element of Fig. 3.29:

- Total resistance in the vasculature is greatest in the arterioles, through a combination of their length and reduced radius without a significant change in total cross-sectional area.

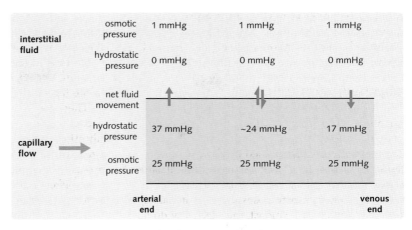

Fig. 3.34 Factors affecting fluid movement across the capillary endothelium. The fall in hydrostatic pressure across the capillary reverses the direction of fluid movement. At the arterial end, there is a net filtration pressure of $(37-25) - (1-0) = 11$ mmHg, forcing fluid out of the capillary. At the venous end, this value becomes $(17-25) - (1-0) = -9$ mmHg, indicating a net filtration pressure drawing fluid back into the capillary (reabsorption).

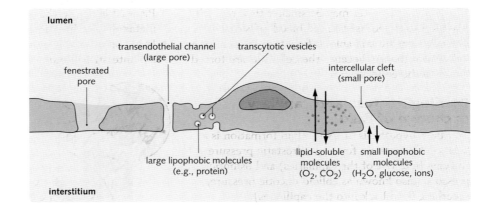

Fig. 3.35 Summary diagram of capillary transport showing the various transport mechanisms.

results if filtration exceeds both reabsorption and the lymphatic system's capacity to remove excess fluid, resulting in an accumulation of fluid in this space.

- In liver disease or severe starvation, plasma protein levels fall, decreasing osmotic pressure. This will drive fluid into the interstitium, leading to edema.
- Capillaries become more permeable to protein when damaged, causing a decrease in plasma osmotic pressure and leading to edema (this process occurs, for example, in the swelling of a sprained joint).

Capillary transport mechanisms

Exchange of solutes generally occurs by diffusion down concentration gradients. The processes involved include:

- Diffusion through the endothelial cell membrane.
- Diffusion through pores and fenestrations in the cell membrane.
- Active transportation by transcytotic vesicles (Fig. 3.35).

Lipid-soluble substances (e.g., oxygen and carbon dioxide) diffuse readily through the endothelial cell membrane of the entire capillary wall.

Pores and fenestrations

Water-soluble substances (e.g., water, glucose, amino acids, ions) diffuse through the many small pores (radii of 4 nm) that constitute the intercellular clefts between endothelial cells. There are also a few large pores for larger molecules, especially in the liver and spleen, where the endothelium is not continuous.

Fenestrated capillaries in exocrine glands have large windows (50-nm radius), which are covered with a mesh of fibers that does not allow molecules larger than 70 kD to pass through. This makes the

55

capillaries more permeable to water but prevents loss of proteins.

In the brain, the endothelial cell junctions have a complex arrangement of fibers that makes them impermeable to lipophobic molecules. This comprises the blood–brain barrier, which tightly controls the neuronal environment of the brain.

Transcytotic vesicles
Some molecules (e.g., proteins) are transported across the endothelial cell by vesicles. This is an active transport process requiring energy.

Lymph and the lymphatic system

Distribution of the lymphatic tissues
Fluid and any proteins and fat globules not reabsorbed into capillaries are brought back into the blood system through the lymphatic system (Fig. 3.36). The network of lymphatic capillaries,

ducts, and lymph nodes unites to form the thoracic duct, which drains into the left subclavian vein.

No lymph drainage exists in the brain or eye, which have their own drainage systems—the cerebrospinal fluid and aqueous humor, respectively.

There are certain specialized areas of lymphatic tissue associated with the immune response:
- Primary lymphoid tissue—thymus and bone marrow.
- Secondary lymphoid tissue—lymph nodes, spleen, and mucosa-associated lymphoid tissue (MALT).

Structure of lymph vessels
Compared with the arterial and venous systems, the lymphatic system is relatively poorly understood. Lymph capillaries are blind ending, thin walled, and usually form a network of tubes of

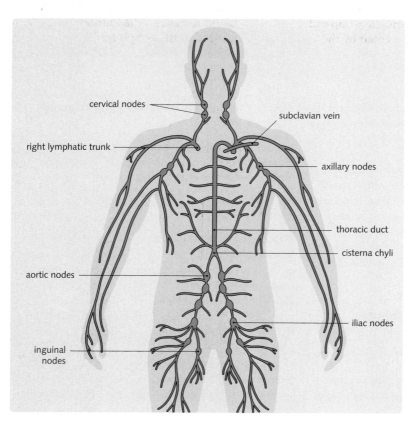

Fig. 3.36 Lymphatic drainage of the body. The lymphatics drain into the left and right subclavian veins.

cervical nodes
subclavian vein
right lymphatic trunk
axillary nodes
thoracic duct
cisterna chyli
aortic nodes
iliac nodes
inguinal nodes

10–50 µm in diameter (see Fig. 3.21). These terminal lymphatics have large endothelial cell junctions, and so they are permeable to plasma proteins and other large molecules. These cell junctions may act like valves, preventing fluid moving back into the interstitium.

Lymph capillaries join together to form collecting vessels, which may contain valves to prevent backflow. Lymph vessels of this size and larger also have smooth muscle in their walls. Afferent vessels drain into a lymph node, where the fluid is presented to the immune system. Some lymph may enter the blood system at these nodes.

Efferent vessels leave the lymph node and enter the cisterna chyli, which acts as a temporary reservoir for chylomicrons from the gut. Eventually, the lymph drains into the large thoracic duct, which drains into the left subclavian vein.

Fluid and proteins are driven into the lymphatic capillaries by the interstitial fluid pressure (possibly aided by lymphatic contraction creating suction). Lymph is moved along the lymphatics by smooth muscle contractions in the vessel wall, which increase with volume, and extrinsic propulsion by the skeletal muscle pump and intestinal peristalsis. Backflow is prevented by the presence of valves.

Role of the lymphatics

The role of the lymphatic system is four-fold:

- Transportation of fluid and proteins. This maintains fluid balance by returning capillary filtrate to the blood.
- Absorption and transport of fat from the gastrointestinal tract. Chylomicrons are tiny fat globules, which are absorbed into intestinal lymph vessels (lacteals).
- Presentation of foreign materials to the immune system. Phagocytosis of particles can occur in the lymph nodes.
- Circulation of lymphocytes. If the immune response is stimulated, lymphocytes can be released from lymph nodes into the lymph to be carried into the blood.

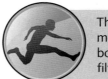

The lymphatics are the mopping-up system of the body, taking up any excess filtrate and returning it to the main circulatory system. They also carry foreign antigens from the blood to cells of the immune system located in the lymph nodes.

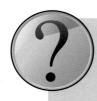

- Describe the functional and anatomic classifications of vessels and how the classifications differ.
- Identify the main vessels of the body and their main branches.
- Explain how the fetal circulation changes at birth.
- Describe the layers of a typical major vessel and their functions.
- List the functions of the vascular endothelium.
- List the factors that affect the contractility of vascular smooth muscle.
- Explain how norepinephrine brings about contraction of vascular smooth muscle.
- Explain how relaxation is brought about in vascular smooth muscle.
- Sketch the pulse waveform. Explain the pulse pressure.
- Describe how to measure blood pressure.
- Define Poiseuille's law.
- Explain the basis for the changes in vascular resistance through the vascular tree and how these changes affect blood pressure and the velocity of blood flow.
- Explain what alters viscosity of blood.
- Explain what affects venous flow.
- Explain how capillaries withstand blood pressure.
- Describe a typical capillary bed and how flow fluctuates.
- Explain Starling's capillary forces and how the movement of water varies within the capillary.
- List the various methods of capillary transport.
- Outline the distribution of the lymph vessels in the body.
- Explain the role of the lymphatic system.

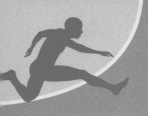

4. Control of the Cardiovascular System

Control of blood vessels

Overview of vascular control

The main function of the vasculature is to deliver metabolic requirements to the tissues of the body. Some tissues have a greater need than others (Fig. 4.1), depending on their function at a given time (e.g., muscles in exercise).

Some tissues can survive without these substrates longer than others (e.g., muscle cells can survive hypoxia for hours, whereas the brain will die within minutes).

Local control mechanisms
Local temperature

This is the main control mechanism in skin. High temperature causes vasodilatation in skin arterioles and veins. In contrast, at temperatures of 12–15°C (55–60°F), vasoconstriction of skin vessels occurs. This appears to be caused by noradrenergic stimulation of α_2-adrenoceptors. Below 12°C, paradoxical cold vasodilatation occurs. Neurotransmitter release is impaired, and vasodilator substances (e.g., prostaglandins) are released.

In most other tissues, vasodilatation occurs in response to cold. This is probably related to the predominance of α_1-receptors in other tissues compared with α_2-receptors in the skin.

Transmural pressure

This is the pressure across the wall of the vessel, and it can be affected by external and internal pressures:

- External pressure. Blood flow is impaired by a high external pressure outside the vessel (e.g., when muscle is contracted or when sitting or kneeling).
- Internal pressure. Initially, raised blood pressure causes the vessel to distend briefly. This causes the smooth muscle to be stretched, producing a contractile response. The vessel becomes constricted, increasing resistance and reducing

Distribution of cardiac output				
Organ	Mass (kg)	Blood flow (mL/min)	Blood flow per 100 g (mL/min/100 g)	Proportion of cardiac output (%)
Brain	1.4	750	54.0	13.9 (18.4)
Heart	0.3	250	84.0	47 (11.6)
Liver	1.5	1500*	100.0*	27.8 (16.1)
Gastrointestinal tract	2.5	1170	46.8	21.7 (16.00)
Kidneys	0.3	1260	420	23.3 (7.2)
Skeletal muscle	31.0	840	2.7	15.6 (20.0)
Skin	3.6	460	12.8	8.6 (4.8)
Rest of body	22.4	340	1.5	6.1 (17.6)
Whole body	63.0	5400	8.6	100 (100)

Fig. 4.1 Distribution of cardiac output to the various systems of the body. Note that the blood flow to the gastrointestinal tract also flows through the liver via the portal circulation. Values for the liver marked * include the portal and arterial circulation to the liver. Values in parentheses denote the percentage of oxygen consumption by the various systems.

flow within the vessel. This is termed the "myogenic response," and it is a mechanism of autoregulation.

Local metabolites

Altered levels of many metabolites cause vasodilatation and increase perfusion of the tissue. These include:

- Hypoxia (i.e., decreased PO_2).
- Acidosis (caused by CO_2 and lactate).
- Adenosine triphosphate (ATP) breakdown products.
- K^+ (from contracting muscle and active brain neurons).
- Increase in osmolarity.

Different tissues are influenced to varying degrees by these factors; for example, coronary vessels react mainly to hypoxia and adenosine, whereas cerebral vessels are influenced by K^+, H^+, and PCO_2.

Cytokines

Cytokines are chemical substances that are produced, secreted, and act as local hormones, producing local responses (e.g., inflammation, hyperemia). They include the following:

- Histamine. This is an inflammatory mediator that causes arteriolar vasodilatation (H_1-receptor mediated). In veins, it causes vasoconstriction and increased permeability (H_2-receptor mediated).
- Bradykinin. This inflammatory mediator causes vasodilatation—nitric oxide (NO)-mediated—and increased vascular permeability (mediated by Ca^{2+}).
- 5-Hydroxytryptamine (5-HT, serotonin). This is found in platelets, the intestinal wall, and the central nervous system. It causes vasoconstriction. Production from platelets contributes significantly to vasoconstriction in response to vessel injury.
- Prostaglandins (PGs). These are inflammatory mediators synthesized from arachidonic acid by cyclooxygenase. They are produced by macrophages, leukocytes, fibroblasts, and endothelium. Their production is inhibited by nonsteroidal anti-inflammatory drugs (NSAIDs) and steroids. PGF causes vasoconstriction; PGE causes vasodilatation, and PGI_2 (prostacyclin) also causes vasodilatation.
- Thromboxane A_2. This is a platelet activator that causes vasoconstriction; it is involved in hemostasis.

- Leukotrienes. These are inflammatory mediators synthesized from arachidonic acid by lipoxygenase. They are produced by leukocytes, and they cause vasoconstriction and increased vascular permeability.
- Platelet-activating factor (PAF). This is an inflammatory mediator that causes vasodilatation, increased vascular permeability, and vasospasm in hypoxic coronary vessels.

Endothelium-dependent relaxation and contraction

When stimulated, the endothelium of arteries and veins produces endothelium-derived relaxing factor (EDRF). EDRF was discovered to be nitric oxide (NO) and is produced in endothelial cells by cleavage from L-arginine by NO synthase. Stimuli include thrombin, bradykinin, substance-P, adenosine diphosphate (ADP), acetylcholine, and histamine.

NO diffuses into smooth muscle cells and activates an intracellular cyclic guanosine monophosphate (cGMP) messenger system, causing relaxation and vasodilatation.

The products of platelet activation stimulate NO release from intact endothelium. This ensures that vasoconstriction only occurs with significant endothelial damage. Healthy endothelium will maintain vessel patency through NO, but injured endothelium will not counteract platelet-initiated vasoconstriction.

Blood flowing through an artery causes shear stress on the endothelial cell. When arterioles dilate to increase tissue perfusion, flow increases in feeder arteries by a process called flow-induced vasodilatation. This process is caused by increased shear stress, increasing NO production.

Vasoconstrictor substances are also produced by the endothelium—endothelin is a powerful vasoconstrictive peptide released in response to stretch, thrombin, and epinephrine. Endothelin acts locally but may have a role in the systemic regulation of blood pressure, and it has been the target for experimental therapeutic agents.

Autoregulation

Autoregulation is the process whereby tissue perfusion remains relatively constant even though blood pressure changes. It also keeps capillary filtration pressure at a stable value.

Flow is proportional to pressure difference divided by resistance. Therefore, to keep flow constant, any pressure change must be opposed by a resistance change. An increase in pressure causes arteriolar vasoconstriction, thereby increasing resistance. A decrease in pressure causes arteriolar vasodilatation and decreases resistance. It takes 30–60 seconds for the effect to take place; so, for example, there is an initial increase in flow with a pressure increase before a steady state is reached.

Autoregulation occurs over a limited pressure range. It is an intrinsic feature of the vessels, and it is independent of nervous control. However, it does not mean that tissue perfusion is constant all the time *in vivo*. Autoregulation can be reset to work at a new level (e.g., an increased sympathetic drive). The mechanisms for autoregulation are:

- Myogenic response. Increased pressure produces constriction of the vessel, opposing the rise in pressure and stabilizing blood flow.
- Vasodilator washout. This is the effect that blood flow has on the concentration of the local vasodilator metabolites. If blood flow increases, these metabolites are washed away faster, causing the vessel to constrict, thereby increasing resistance and decreasing flow back to normal.
- In the heart, any increase in coronary arterial pressure causes a rise in tissue PO_2, leading to vasoconstriction; this autoregulates heart blood flow.

Metabolic hyperemia

Metabolic (or functional/active) hyperemia is the increase in blood flow that occurs in exercising muscle and secreting exocrine glands when their metabolic rate increases. The production of local vasodilator metabolites leads to vasodilatation and causes vascular resistance to fall.

Flow-induced vasodilatation causes the main artery to dilate. Ascending dilatation from the arterioles to the feeder arteries leads to dilatation of the whole arterial tree supplying the tissue.

Blood flow in contracting muscle is increased in the resting phase. In the heart, the increase in metabolic rate causes a drop in tissue PO_2, leading to vasodilatation.

Reactive hyperemia

Reactive (or postischemic) hyperemia is the increase in blood flow that occurs after supply to a tissue has been temporarily interrupted.

Reactive hyperemia enables resupply to ischemic tissue as quickly as possible. The myogenic response is the predominant mechanism for brief occlusions, dilating the downstream vessels in preparation for the return of blood flow. In more prolonged occlusions, vasodilator metabolites accumulate, and these play a significant role. Prostaglandins also aid this process.

Reactive hyperemia is temporary, and it decays exponentially. A plateau of hyperemia may precede decay in prolonged occlusions. In some tissues (e.g., the heart), there is an oversupply of blood and oxygen compared with the deficit during the temporary interruption to flow.

Ischemic reperfusion injury

When blood flow to a tissue is interrupted for a prolonged period, reactive hyperemia is impaired.

Reperfusion of ischemic tissue results in superoxide ($O_2^{-\bullet}$) and hydroxide ($OH^\bullet$) radical formation. These damage the tissue and vessel wall, causing further occlusion. Damage is exacerbated by an increase in K^+ and tissue acidosis. Reperfused cells have an impaired plasmalemmal barrier to Ca^{2+} ions, which flow into the cell in an unrestricted way, causing calcium overload damage.

It is thought that reperfusion injury exacerbates damage to the myocardium, intestine, and brain following ischemia.

 Most locally produced substances increase blood flow because the tissue wants to wash them away (e.g., lactate and adenosine are waste products of metabolism, which need to be removed).

Nervous control

Fig. 4.2 gives an overview of nervous control of the vasculature.

Sympathetic vasoconstrictor nerves

Sympathetic vasoconstrictor nerves innervate the vascular smooth muscle of the resistance and capacitance vessels. A basal level of activity of these nerves is responsible for vessel tone at rest. The neurotransmitter released is norepinephrine, which acts on α_1-receptors on vascular smooth muscle, causing contraction. When there is an increase in sympathetic drive:

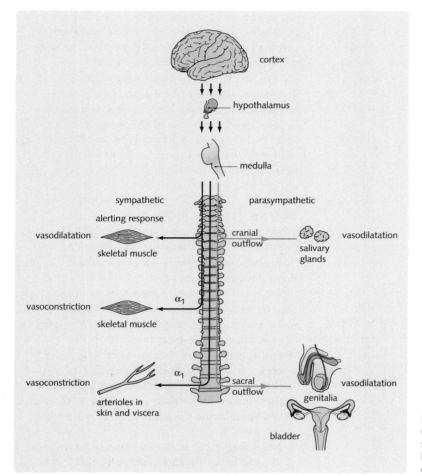

Fig. 4.2 Overview of nervous control of the vasculature. The sympathetic tracts are shown on the left and the parasympathetic tracts on the right.

- Vasoconstriction decreases local blood flow.
- Venoconstriction decreases local blood volume.
- Arteriolar constriction decreases capillary pressure, leading to greater resorption of fluid from the interstitium back into the blood.

If there is an increase in sympathetic activity throughout the body, total peripheral resistance and cardiac output increase. This constitutes the basis of the sympathetic response to hemorrhage.

A decrease in sympathetic activity causes vasodilatation and venodilatation.

Sympathetic vasodilator nerves

Some tissues (skeletal muscle and sweat glands) are also innervated by sympathetic vasodilator nerves. In skeletal muscle, vascular bed stimulation by these nerves (which use acetylcholine as the neurotransmitter and act on muscarinic receptors)

causes vasodilatation. Stimulation only occurs as part of an "alerting response," and it is initiated in the forebrain without any brainstem influence. The vasodilator effect is only temporary, and it plays no role in blood pressure regulation. Stimulation of these nerves in sweat glands—probably involving vasoactive intestinal peptide (VIP) as neurotransmitter—produces sweating and cutaneous vasodilatation. In theory, these nerves would prepare the organism for exercise by increasing muscle blood flow before any activity is initiated.

Parasympathetic vasodilator nerves

Parasympathetic vasodilator nerves innervate the blood vessels of:

- The head.
- Salivary glands.
- Pancreas.

- Gastrointestinal mucosa.
- Genitalia.
- Bladder.

The effect of these nerves on the total peripheral resistance is small because of their limited innervation. Their postganglionic neurons release acetylcholine, which relaxes vascular smooth muscle.

In some tissues (e.g., the pancreas), VIP may be the main neurotransmitter. Vasodilatation occurs in the arteries and arterioles of these vascular beds.

In the erectile tissue of the penis and clitoris, it is parasympathetic and nitroxidergic vasodilatation that fill the corpus sinuses with blood, causing erection.

Nitroxidergic vasodilator nerves

Nitric oxide has recently been recognized as a neurotransmitter, both in the central and peripheral nervous system. Such neurons are referred to as nitrergic or nitroxidergic. They act on smooth muscle cells, causing relaxation. Nitrergic innervation has so far been found in the regulation of muscle tone in the gut and in sexual arousal in the male and female genitalia.

At present, pharmacologic manipulation of nitrergic transmission is limited to the use of sildenafil (Viagra) and similar agents in the treatment of male impotence. Sildenafil acts by selective inhibition of the phosphodiesterase present in smooth muscle of the genital vessels. This potentiates the effect of nitrergic stimulation (phosphodiesterase enzymes break up the cGMP that mediates the relaxation in response to NO). Sildenafil should not be given to hypotensive patients, nor combined with other forms of systemic nitrate treatment due to the risk of syncope.

Hormonal control

Although short-term, immediate regulation of the vasculature is under the control of the sympathetic nervous system, circulating hormones play an important intermediate role in controlling blood pressure.

Epinephrine

The catecholamines epinephrine (EPI) and norepinephrine (NE) are considered neurohumoral regulators because they are released in response to nervous stimulation, but they can also act as circulating agents. Epinephrine is the primary catecholamine released from the adrenal medulla, whereas norepinephrine is the primary catecholamine released from nerve terminals. This difference is due to the fact that the adrenal medulla is the primary source of the enzyme phenyethanolamine-n-methyl transferase, which converts NE to EPI. At rest, plasma levels of EPI and NE are 0.1–0.5 nmol/L and 0.5–3.0 nmol/L, respectively. Plasma levels of NE are higher because of "spillover" from sympathetic nerve terminals and the relatively low level of adrenal medullary stimulation. During times of high sympathetic activity (exercise, hypotension, fight-or-flight situations), however, the adrenal medulla is stimulated, and plasma levels of both catecholamines may increase substantially.

Both hormones are β_1-adrenoceptor agonists, so they increase heart rate and contractility of the myocardium. Both hormones cause vasoconstriction in most tissues via α-receptors:

- Epinephrine causes vasoconstriction in most organs (especially skin), but vasodilatation in skeletal muscle, myocardium, and liver because there are more β_2-receptors in these latter tissues, and epinephrine has a higher affinity for these receptors.
- Norepinephrine usually causes vasoconstriction because it has a higher affinity for α-receptors.

Adrenal gland stimulation results predominantly in epinephrine release. Effects on the heart include increased contractility, stroke volume, and heart rate. Blood pressure rises as a result, since the vasodilatory effects of epinephrine do not fully counteract the vasoconstrictor effects combined with the increased cardiac output.

Vasopressin (antidiuretic hormone)

Antidiuretic hormone (ADH) is a peptide produced in the hypothalamus and released from the posterior pituitary into the bloodstream. A rise in plasma osmolarity is the main stimulus for secretion. Falling blood pressure and volume are also stimuli, but to a lesser degree.

ADH promotes water retention by the kidney. High levels of ADH cause vasoconstriction in most tissues. In the brain and heart, NO-mediated vasodilatation occurs. This ensures preferential supply to the brain and heart in hypovolemia.

Renin–angiotensin–aldosterone

Renin is an enzyme produced by the juxtaglomerular cells of the kidney. It converts angiotensinogen (from the liver) to angiotensin I (Fig. 4.3). Renin production is increased by:

- A fall in afferent arterial pressure to the glomeruli.
- Increased sympathetic activity.
- Decreased Na^+ delivery to the macula densa.

Angiotensin-converting enzyme (ACE) converts angiotensin I to the peptide angiotensin II (see Fig. 4.3), which has the following actions:

- Increases aldosterone secretion from the adrenal cortex.
- Causes vasoconstriction at high concentration by acting directly on vascular smooth muscle, initiating release of norepinephrine from sympathetic nerve terminals, and increasing central sympathetic drive in the brainstem.
- Increases cardiac contractility.

Aldosterone increases salt and water retention by renal tubules.

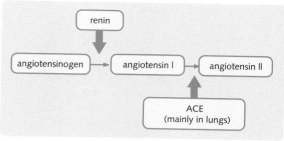

Fig. 4.3 Formation of angiotensin II. Angiotensinogen is secreted by the liver, acted on by renin (secreted by the kidney), and finally converted to the active angiotensin II by angiotensin-converting enzyme (ACE).

In addition to converting angiotensin I to angiotensin II, ACE is also responsible for the breakdown of bradykinin, a vasodilator peptide. Although this may play a minor role in the hypotensive actions of ACE inhibitors, it is responsible for one of their common toxicities. In addition to its vasodilatory actions, bradykinin is an irritant, and its local accumulation leads to the cough and sore throat often associated with ACE inhibitor therapy (remember, ACE is located primarily in the lung).

Atrial natriuretic peptide

In response to high cardiac filling pressure, specialized myocytes in the atria secrete atrial natriuretic peptide (ANP). ANP increases the excretion of salt and water by renal tubules. It also has a slight vasodilating effect.

Ventricles similarly secrete brain natriuretic peptide (BNP), which increases in heart failure. Levels of BNP may be used as a blood test for heart failure.

Cardiovascular receptors and central control

The cardiovascular system is regulated and controlled by the brain through autonomic nerves (Fig. 4.4).

Remember: **Pressure** is the regulated variable in the cardiovascular system. It seems simple, but many students forget this and get confused on the national boards.

Arterial baroreceptors and the baroreflex

Arterial baroreceptors (stretch receptors) are located in the carotid sinus and aortic arch. They play a key role in short-term blood pressure control, and they respond to stretch of the vessel wall. They continually produce impulses at normal vessel wall tone. Increased stretch (due to increased pressure) increases firing frequency, whereas decreased stretch decreases the firing rate.

The impulse that the baroreceptor generates is carried to the medulla by the glossopharyngeal nerves (carotid sinus) and the vagus nerves (aortic arch).

At the medulla, there is an interaction with the other central pathways. An increased firing rate causes the medulla to:

- Increase vagal (parasympathetic) drive.
- Decrease sympathetic drive.

This results in a decrease in heart rate. Contractility is probably not affected to a great degree. It also

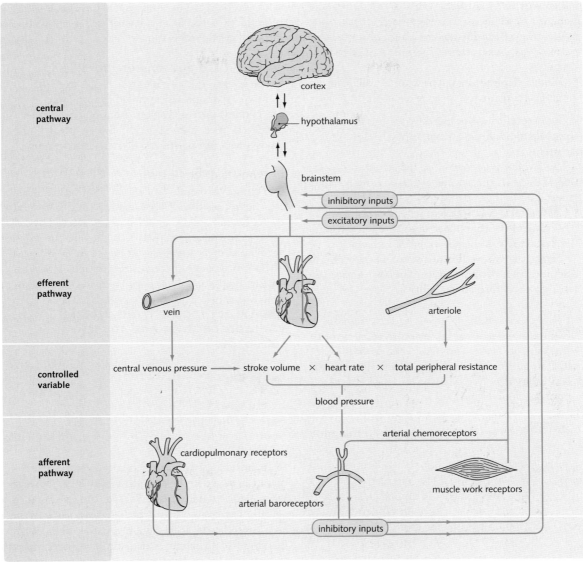

Fig. 4.4 Overview of the central control of the circulation (adapted from *Introducing Cardiovascular Physiology* by Levick R, New York, Butterworth–Heinemann, 1995).

causes a fall in total peripheral resistance. These measures all serve to reduce blood pressure back to normal. The baroreceptors are said to buffer the blood pressure in the short term.

When the baroreceptor is unloaded (stretch is reduced), the firing rate to the medulla is reduced. The effect is to decrease vagal and increase sympathetic drive. This results in:
- Increased heart rate and contractility.
- Peripheral vasoconstriction and venoconstriction.

- Catecholamine secretion.
- Increased renin secretion.

The effect is to increase cardiac output, total peripheral resistance, and the circulating volume, all of which serve to return blood pressure to normal.

The baroreflex is very rapid (<1 second for bradycardia to occur), and it is very important in acute hypotension and hemorrhage and in cardiac adjustments to postural change.

The sensitivity of the arterial baroreceptors to a change in blood pressure is decreased by:

- Age. The compliance of the arterial wall falls with age, which means there is less stretch of the arterial walls.
- Chronic hypertension. The arterial wall loses its distensibility.

The baroreflex is inhibited by stimulation of the hypothalamic defense area in fight-or-flight situations.

The level of blood pressure that the baroreceptor takes as normal (the set point) can be reset by central or peripheral processes:

- Central resetting. In exercise, the rise in blood pressure that occurs does not cause a bradycardia because there has been a central influence to operate the baroreflex at a new higher level. The neurons that drive inspiration inhibit cardiac vagal nerves, therefore blocking baroreceptor impulses and causing a decreased vagal drive.
- Peripheral resetting. Chronic hypertension or hypotension leads to the set point being reset to this new pressure. This allows the baroreflex to operate in its optimal range. This is also why the baroreflex is not very useful for long-term blood pressure homeostasis.

 Baroreceptors and the baroreceptor reflex are very important for **short-term** regulation of blood pressure. Their role is a common exam question.

Cardiopulmonary receptors

There are many cardiopulmonary receptors connected to afferent fibers innervating the heart, great veins, and pulmonary artery. Overall, stimulation of these receptors causes bradycardia, vasodilatation, and hypotension. There are three main classes of receptor with differing functions—venoatrial stretch receptors, unmyelinated mechanoreceptor fibers, and chemosensitive fibers.

Venoatrial stretch receptors

These are branched nerve endings located where the great veins join the atria. They are connected to large myelinated vagal fibers. Stimulation produces a reflex tachycardia by selectively increasing sympathetic drive to the pacemaker. This is often referred to as the Bainbridge reflex. There is also an increase in salt and water excretion.

Unmyelinated mechanoreceptor fibers

These are present in both atria and in the left ventricle. Afferent fibers travel in vagal and sympathetic nerves. Large distension stimulates these receptors, causing an inhibitory effect. Reflex bradycardia and peripheral vasodilatation occur.

Chemosensitive fibers

Some unmyelinated vagal and sympathetic afferents are chemosensitive. They are stimulated in response to bradykinin and other substances released by an ischemic myocardium. It is thought that the pain of angina and myocardial infarction is caused by these fibers. Stimulation increases respiration as well as causing bradycardia and peripheral vasodilatation.

Excitatory inputs from arterial chemoreceptors and muscle receptors

Chemoreceptors are located in the carotid and aortic bodies. They are nerve terminals whose excitation is increased by hypoxia, hypercapnia, and acidosis of arterial blood (see *Crash Course: Respiratory System*). Their fibers travel with afferent baroreceptor fibers in the glossopharyngeal and vagus nerves.

At normal gas tensions, chemoreceptors are mainly involved in the control of breathing. However, when their excitation is increased, they respond by causing a sympathetically mediated vasoconstriction and a mild bradycardia. The respiratory chemoreflex increases tidal volume, which stimulates lung stretch receptors. This causes a marked tachycardia and a modest vasodilatation. Overall, the heart rate and blood pressure increase to enhance perfusion. The chemoreflex plays an important role in asphyxia, severe hemorrhage, and hypotension, where the chemoreceptors are excited by the reduced metabolite supply (and blood pressure is below baroreceptor range).

Skeletal muscle produces a reflex cardiovascular response to exercise. This is stimulated by metaboloreceptors (activated by K^+ and H^+) and mechanoreceptors (activated by pressure and tension). The excitation travels through small nerve fibers (groups III and IV). The reflex produces tachycardia, increased myocardial contractility, and vasoconstriction in other vascular beds. This allows greater perfusion of the exercising muscle. This is termed the "exercise pressor response," and it is greater in static exercise.

Central pathways

The central pathways that influence the cardiovascular system have only been partly explained. They involve a complex interaction between the medulla, hypothalamus, cerebellum, and cortex.

Medulla

It used to be thought that there was a specific vasomotor center in the medulla. Now it is thought that there are complex signals between the hypothalamus, cortex, and cerebellum as well as signals within the vasomotor center of the medulla. In general, the rostral ventrolateral medulla is responsible for the sympathetic outflow, whereas the nucleus ambiguous is responsible for the parasympathetic outflow; these two areas control vessel tone and heart rate.

Information from baroreceptors is received (at the nucleus tractus solitarius) by the medulla, and it is relayed to the hypothalamus. Medullary autonomic control is also influenced by hypothalamic activity.

Hypothalamus

This contains four areas of interest:
- Depressor area. This can produce the baroreflex, but it is not vital for the reflex to occur.
- Defense area. This is responsible for the alerting response and the fight-or-flight response. It therefore plays a role in governing sympathetic outflow.
- Temperature-regulating area. This controls cutaneous vascular tone and sweating.
- Vasopressin-secreting area. This produces vasopressin, which travels through nerve axons to the pituitary.

Cerebellum

The cerebellum's primary role is muscle coordination. During exercise, the cerebellum helps to coordinate the response to exercise.

Cortex

The cortex may initiate or suppress many of the cardiovascular responses. The effects of fear and emotion on the vasculature probably have a cortical influence.

Regulation of circulation in individual tissues

Blood flow rates in various circulations are given in Fig. 4.5.

Coronary circulation

Myocardial oxygen demand is very high, being about 8 mL O_2/min/100 g. During exercise, cardiac work can increase fivefold, thereby increasing oxygen demand. Since the heart extracts nearly all the oxygen present in the blood perfusing it, demand can only be met by increasing flow.

Oxygen transport is aided by the high capillary density (large area and decreased distance for exchange) and the presence of myoglobin. There is a high oxygen extraction from the capillaries (>60%) even at rest, resulting in low oxygen levels in coronary venous blood.

Blood flow is mainly controlled by tissue PO_2. Low PO_2 produces a metabolic hyperemia. Metabolic vasodilatation can be partly opposed by sympathetic α_1-noradrenergic vasoconstriction.

Flow rate in various circulations		
Circulation	Basal flow rate (mL/min/100 g)	Maximum flow rate (minimum) (mL/min/100 g)
Coronary	80	400
Phasic (white, fast) skeletal muscle	3	200 (on exercise)
Tonic (red, slow) skeletal muscle	15	200 (on exercise)
Cutaneous	10–20 (at 27°C)	200
Brain Gray matter	55 100	– –
Renal	400	–
Liver GIT	85 40	150 (after food) 80 (after food)

Fig. 4.5 Resting and maximum blood flow rates in the various circulations (GIT, gastrointestinal tract).

Epinephrine acts on β₂-receptors in coronary smooth muscle to dilate the vessels and increase blood flow.

Coronary arteries are functional end-arteries with few cross-connections between them. They are at risk of being blocked by thrombosis, causing ischemia. There are, however, some collateral vessels, which may delay the onset of ischemia. During systole, coronary artery branches in the myocardium are compressed, effectively reducing blood flow. Flow is fully restored only during diastole (Fig. 4.6).

Skeletal muscle

Oxygen and nutrient delivery to the muscle cells must increase with exercise. Removal of waste products and heat must also be increased during exercise.

Skeletal muscle makes up 40% of body mass. Its vasculature contributes significantly to vascular resistance and, therefore, affects blood pressure homeostasis.

Phasically active muscle consists of white fibers (e.g., gastrocnemius). Postural muscles (e.g., soleus) are tonically active red fibers, and they have a greater capillary density.

Sympathetic vasoconstrictor nerve reflexes controlled by baroreceptors play a major role in controlling flow. In hypovolemia, for example, vasoconstriction can reduce flow in skeletal muscle to one fifth of its resting value.

During exercise, metabolic vasodilatation is the dominant mechanism for increasing flow. Epinephrine causes vasodilatation by acting on smooth-muscle β₂-receptors; this is aided by the actions of local metabolites.

In contrast to the myocardium, at rest only 25% of the oxygen in the blood is extracted. In severe exercise, this extraction can be increased considerably. Extraction is aided by the presence of myoglobin.

The skeletal muscle pump aids venous return to the heart. This lowers venous pressure in the limbs. The pressure difference from the arterial to venous circulations increases. Thus, the perfusion pressure is increased, driving blood flow.

Blood flow is impaired during contraction. If contraction is sustained, then the fibers will become hypoxic. Lactate will accumulate causing pain, and strength will be rapidly lost.

An increase in the capillary filtration rate can lead to a fall in plasma volume.

Cutaneous circulation

The skin has a low metabolic requirement, and its vasculature is mainly involved in the regulation of the internal core body temperature.

Specific areas of the skin have arteriovenous anastomoses (Fig. 4.7). These exposed areas have a high surface area to volume ratio and include the fingers, toes, palms, soles of the feet, lips, nose, and ears. These anastomoses are controlled by sympathetic vasoconstrictor nerves. In turn, the sympathetic activity is controlled via the brainstem by the temperature-regulating area in

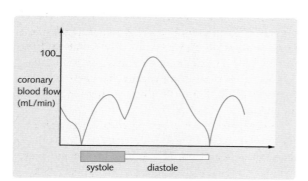

Fig. 4.6 Coronary blood flow during the cardiac cycle. Note that maximal blood flow is during diastole.

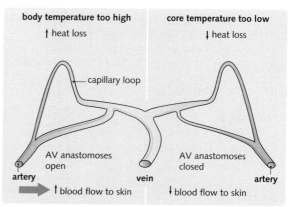

Fig. 4.7 Temperature control by arteriovenous (AV) anastomoses.

the hypothalamus. The nerves controlling sweating are also controlled in the same way—when the core body temperature is too high, sympathetic drive is reduced, and the arteriovenous anastomoses dilate.

Skin temperature is very variable, because it is influenced by ambient temperature. It has a direct effect on cutaneous vascular tone:
• Local heating causes vasodilatation.
• Local cooling causes vasoconstriction.

Paradoxical cold vasodilatation occurs in acral areas (the extremities) on prolonged exposure to cold. After the initial vasoconstriction, vasodilatation occurs. This is thought to be because the cold impairs sympathetic vasoconstriction. This phenomenon prevents skin damage in such exposure.

Hypotension causes a neural and hormonal (angiotensin, ADH, and epinephrine) vasoconstriction of skin vessels. This produces the cold skin seen in shock.

Exercise causes vasoconstriction of the skin initially, but this can become a dilatation if the core temperature rises.

Emotion can produce a hyperemic response in the skin (blushing) and the gastric and colonic mucosa.

Compression of the skin for long periods (e.g., when sitting) impairs blood flow. Reactive hyperemia and the skin's high tolerance to hypoxia prevent ischemic damage. Restlessness (i.e., the desire to move position) also plays a major role, possibly stimulated by local metabolites and pain receptors. In certain patients, however, failure to move or be moved can lead to necrosis in compressed areas (bed sores, decubitus).

In hot weather, cutaneous vasodilatation can lower central venous pressure. This can lead to fainting (e.g., a soldier while standing to attention on a hot day must use his skeletal muscle pump to maintain venous pressure; otherwise, he will suddenly faint).

Cerebral circulation

Gray matter has a high oxygen consumption (7 mL O_2/min/100 g). Because gray matter has little tolerance to hypoxia, consciousness is lost after a few seconds of ischemia.

The cerebral circulation primarily uses local metabolites to adjust blood flow and meet local demand. This is accomplished mainly by an increase in interstitial K^+, causing metabolic hyperemia.

In young people, the circle of Willis enables blood supply to be maintained if one carotid artery is occluded. These anastomoses linking the supply arteries together are less effective in the elderly. There is a high capillary density, similar in size to that in the myocardium. The presence of a blood–brain barrier tightly controls the neuronal environment. Lipid-soluble molecules can diffuse freely, but ionic solutes cannot.

The brain can control cardiac output and vascular resistance of other tissues through autonomic nerves. Cerebral perfusion is maintained at the expense of other tissues when required.

There is good autoregulation of the cerebral blood flow, but this fails when pressure falls below 50 mmHg.

Cerebral vessels are very sensitive to arterial PCO_2:
• Hypercapnia causes vasodilatation (Fig. 4.8).
• Hypocapnia causes vasoconstriction.

Reduction in arterial PCO_2 through hyperventilation can lead to cerebral vasoconstriction and even transient unconsciousness. Cerebral vessels do not participate in baroreflex vasoconstriction.

Pulmonary circulation

The entire output of the right ventricle enters the pulmonary circulation. A separate bronchial circulation from the aorta meets the metabolic needs of the bronchi.

There is a very high capillary density and very thin blood–alveolar surface to maximize gaseous exchange. Gas exchange in the lung is flow limited (i.e., a rise in blood flow increases the rate of oxygen uptake).

Pulmonary arteries and arterioles are shorter, thinner walled, and more easily distensible than systemic vessels so that pulmonary vascular resistance is very low with a low pulmonary arterial pressure (22/8 mmHg). There is no autoregulation of blood flow, although the pulmonary vessels still respond to systemic mediators (e.g., epinephrine).

Low capillary pressure means that there is no filtration of fluid into the alveoli in healthy individuals.

In the upright person, mean arterial pressure at the apex of the lung is about 3 mmHg, and at the base it is about 21 mmHg. At the level of the heart, the mean pressure is 15 mmHg. At the lung base, high pressure causes the thin-walled vessels to distend and blood flow to increase (Fig. 4.8). At the apex, flow primarily occurs during systole, because the diastolic pressure may be insufficient to open the vessels.

The ventilation–perfusion ratio governs the efficiency of oxygen transfer. Although ventilation is greater at the base than at the apex, the difference is not as great as the difference in flow. This implies that the ventilation–perfusion ratio is higher at the apex than at the base, and this mismatch impairs efficiency.

General hypoxia causes pulmonary hypertension. Poorly ventilated areas become poorly perfused because of hypoxic vasoconstriction. This mechanism helps to optimize ventilation–perfusion ratios.

Renal circulation

Renal blood flow is autoregulated over a certain range of blood pressure, which allows a near-constant glomerular filtration rate. Autoregulation fails in severe hypotension (prerenal failure).

The body is very good at diverting blood flow to where it is needed. However, some circulations (e.g., cerebral and renal) are special in that their blood flow is usually preserved at the expense of others.

Mesenteric circulation

The hyperemia associated with the arrival of food (termed "postprandial hyperemia") is caused by:
- Local hormones (e.g., gastrin and cholecystokinin).
- Digestion products (e.g., glucose and fatty acids).
- Increased vagal activity.

The rise in mesenteric/splanchnic blood flow produces a tachycardia and, therefore, an increase in cardiac output of 1 L/min. There is also vasoconstriction in skeletal muscle vascular beds. There is normally no significant change in blood pressure.

Coordinated cardiovascular responses

Cardiovascular response to posture

When moving from supine to standing (orthostasis), the effect of gravity on venous blood causes venous pooling in the legs. There is a fall in intrathoracic blood volume. This leads to decreased cardiac filling and, therefore, decreased stroke volume. This leads to a fall in systemic arterial pressure. This is usually corrected immediately by the baroreflex, but it can cause a transient hypotension, even in healthy individuals. This happens especially when there is already peripheral vasodilatation in a warm environment.

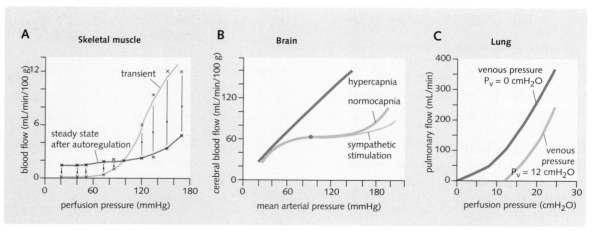

Fig. 4.8 Pressure–flow curves for (A) skeletal muscle, (B) brain vasculature, and (C) lung tissue. A. One line shows transient flow after altering perfusion pressure; the other line shows steady state achieved by autoregulation. B. Autoregulation at normal arterial PCO_2 and the effect of hypercapnia. C. The airway pressure was constant at $4 \, cmH_2O$. Increasing perfusion pressure increases pulmonary flow due to vascular distension and opening of some closed venous vessels. This increase in flow is less marked when venous pressure is above airway pressure.

The baroreceptors and cardiopulmonary receptors react by decreasing their firing rate. This increases sympathetic and decreases parasympathetic outflow, resulting in increased heart rate and contractility. In addition, peripheral vasoconstriction increases total peripheral resistance to bring blood pressure back toward normal. Venoconstriction reduces venous pooling and helps to restore venous return. The net effect of all these changes is maintenance of blood pressure adequate to maintain cerebral perfusion and consciousness. Failure of these mechanisms is associated with postural or orthostatic hypotension (i.e., fainting upon standing). To test this response, it is important to measure blood pressure in both the lying and standing positions.

With prolonged standing, capillary filtration in the legs increases because of venous pooling and the associated elevated venous pressure. This can cause a drop in plasma volume, especially if it is combined with water loss secondary to sweating in a hot environment. Vasopressin and aldosterone (via activation of the renin-angiotensin-aldosterone system) reduce salt and water excretion in an attempt to restore plasma volume. The overall effect is to maintain arterial pressure and ensure adequate tissue perfusion.

Valsalva maneuver

This is a forced expiration against a closed glottis. This commonly occurs when coughing, defecating, and lifting heavy weights. It produces a raised intrathoracic pressure (Fig. 4.9).

This maneuver is a useful test of baroreceptor competence. If the pressure fall in phase 2 continues and there is no bradycardia in phase 4, then the baroreflex is being interrupted, leading to postural hypotension.

Cardiovascular response to exercise

Initial requirements during exercise are:
- Increased gaseous exchange in the pulmonary circulation.
- Increased blood flow to the working muscle.
- Stable blood pressure.

Cardiac output and oxygen uptake

All other factors being unchanged, cardiac output is increased by increases in heart rate or stroke volume (Fig. 4.10):
- Increased heart rate can be caused by sympathetic stimulation or decreased vagal inhibition.
- Stroke volume can be increased by increased cardiac filling (due to skeletal muscle pump and splanchnic vasoconstriction), increased contractility (due to sympathetic stimulation), or a fall in peripheral resistance (due to skeletal muscle vasodilatation).

In upright exercise, stroke volume plays the main role in increasing output. In supine exercise, heart rate increases mainly account for the increased output. Stroke volume increases only at low work rates.

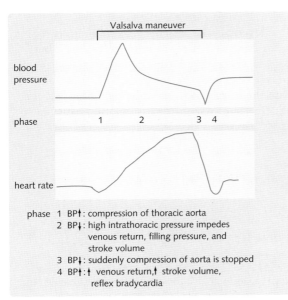

Fig. 4.9 Response to the Valsalva maneuver (BP, blood pressure).

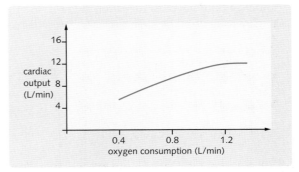

Fig. 4.10 Relationship between cardiac output and oxygen consumption in the whole body. It shows a linear increase of cardiac output with oxygen consumption produced by increased heart rate and stroke volume.

Changes in blood flow to active muscle

Blood flow to active muscle increases with exercise. Hyperemia can be as much as 40 times normal flow, and it is caused by:
- Metabolic vasodilatation.
- Increased pressure gradient by skeletal muscle pump in upright exercise.
- Capillary recruitment by dilatation of terminal arterioles.

The alerting response caused by anticipation of exercise (e.g., at the start of a race) causes an initial sympathetically mediated vasodilatation.

Changes in blood flow in other tissues

Coronary blood flow increases with the increase in cardiac work. Cutaneous vessels initially contract to maintain blood pressure, but they dilate if core temperature rises. Vasoconstriction in the renal, splanchnic, and nonactive muscle vascular beds helps to maintain blood pressure.

Blood pressure during static and dynamic exercise

In dynamic (alternately contracting and relaxing) exercise, the diastolic pressure hardly changes, although the pulse pressure rises (Fig. 4.11). The increase in pressure in static exercise is caused by the exercise pressor response, which is mediated by receptors in the muscle.

Initiation of the response to exercise

The exact causes of the changes in autonomic activity during exercise are not known. Two hypotheses are prevalent:
- The central command hypothesis. This postulates that as the cerebral cortex initiates contraction of muscle, it also instructs the autonomic nerves of the brainstem to increase heart rate. Baroreflex

resetting to a higher value may also be linked to this theory.
- The peripheral reflex hypothesis. The nerve receptors in working muscle are excited by the presence of chemical stimulants, and they cause a reflex sympathetic response, increasing cardiac output and pressure.

It is likely that the central command hypothesis produces the initial tachycardia and vagal suppression. The peripheral reflex hypothesis may account for the slower increase in cardiac output and peripheral vasoconstriction.

Cardiovascular response to training

This is most important in the long-distance or endurance athlete. Training causes improvements in oxygen transport rate and changes in cardiac structure and function. Causes of improved oxygen delivery and extraction are:
- New capillaries formed in skeletal muscle.
- More muscle mitochondria closer to capillaries.
- Increased muscle myoglobin concentration.

Changes in cardiac structure and function are:
- Thicker ventricular wall.
- Increased myocardial vascularity.
- Increased ventricular cavity size.

Stroke volume is much higher because of the cardiac changes. Most athletes have a resting bradycardia, but because of the increased stroke volume, the resting cardiac output is the same.

In exercise, the athlete's maximum heart rate is the same as that for an untrained subject, but because the athlete starts at a lower value, a much greater change can be achieved. This, coupled with the increased stroke volume, means that the athlete can increase cardiac output up to as much as 35 L/min.

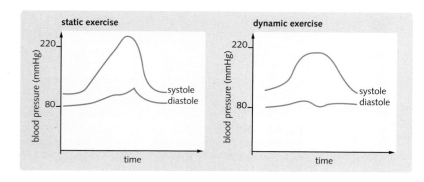

Fig. 4.11 Blood pressure during static and dynamic exercise. Diastolic pressure rises in static exercise, but it remains relatively constant in dynamic exercise. The cardiac work is greater for equivalent static than for dynamic exercise.

Diving reflex

The diving reflex occurs when cold water touches the facial receptors of the trigeminal nerve. The body is expecting a dive into water and a period of submersion. The limited oxygen must be preferentially diverted to the heart and brain. There are three reflexes involved:

- Apnea—Arterial chemoreceptors are triggered as asphyxia develops.
- Bradycardia—caused by intense vagal inhibition of the pacemaker.
- Peripheral vasoconstriction—occurs in the splanchnic, renal, and skeletal muscle vascular beds. The strong, sympathetically mediated vasoconstriction overwhelms any metabolic dilatation that may occur in active muscle.

In marine mammals, the diving reflex is much stronger, and coupled with their larger store of oxygen and myoglobin, this enables them to survive submerged for longer periods.

Syncope

Syncope (fainting or vasovagal attack) is a sudden, transient loss of consciousness as a result of impaired cerebral perfusion. It is caused by a drop in cerebral blood flow to less than half its normal value.

It may be initiated by a pathophysiologic cause (e.g., orthostasis or severe hypovolemia) or by psychological stress (e.g., fear, pain, or horror). In psychogenic fainting, there is often a prefaint period of tachycardia, cutaneous vasoconstriction, hyperventilation, and sweating. A vasovagal faint proceeds as follows:

1. A sudden increase in vagal inhibition leads to bradycardia.
2. Peripheral vasodilatation results due to decreased sympathetic drive.
3. This causes a fall in blood pressure, reducing cerebral blood flow.
4. Loss of consciousness results within seconds.

The cause of the sudden changes is unknown. In psychogenic fainting, it could be a primitive "playing dead" response. In hypovolemic fainting, it could be triggered by mechanoreceptors in the near-empty left ventricle.

The person who has fainted ends up in the supine position. This raises the intrathoracic blood volume and the filling pressure. Coupled with the baroreflex, this then increases cardiac output and arterial pressure. Consciousness is restored in about 2 minutes.

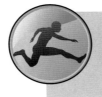 To understand the cardiovascular responses, first decide what has changed, and then think how the body might restore the status quo.

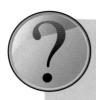

- List the mechanisms involved in the local control of blood flow.
- Explain how nitric oxide is involved in regulating blood flow and vessel diameter.
- Explain how autoregulation is brought about. Define its importance.
- Explain the role of the sympathetic vasoconstrictor nerves in vascular control.
- Explain how and where vasodilator nerves (sympathetic and parasympathetic) operate.
- Identify the principal vasoactive hormones and their effect on the vasculature.
- Explain the baroreflex and how it is elicited.
- List the roles of venoatrial stretch receptors and mechanoreceptors.
- Explain the effects the chemosensitive receptors have on the cardiovascular system.
- Identify the areas of the brain that influence central control.
- With regard to the specialized regulation of the vascular system in different organs:
  - Explain the average resting flow in each organ.
  - Explain how the regulation of flow within that organ relates to its function.
  - Explain how each organ responds to its special circumstances.
- Explain how orthostasis affects cardiac output. Identify the reflexes involved in maintaining blood pressure.
- Explain how the Valsalva maneuver affects the heart and blood pressure. Explain what it can tell us.
- Describe the changes that occur in exercise and how they are brought about.
- Explain how and why there are differences in the response to static and dynamic exercise.
- Explain how the physiology of a top athlete differs from that of the general populace.
- Describe the diving reflex.
- Explain why fainting occurs. Identify the receptors and reflexes involved in the different causes.

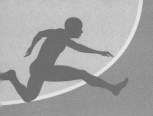

5. The Cardiovascular System in Disease

Shock and hemorrhage

Shock
Definition
Shock is an acute failure of the cardiovascular system to adequately perfuse the tissues of the body.

There are four major shock categories, depending on the causative factor:
- Hypovolemic shock.
- Septicemic shock.
- Cardiogenic shock.
- Anaphylactic shock.

Symptoms
The symptoms of shock are:
- Faintness, light-headedness, dizziness.
- Sweating.
- Reduced level of consciousness.

Signs
The classic signs of shock are:
- Pale, cold, clammy skin caused by cutaneous vasoconstriction in an effort to conserve blood flow to the vital organs and sweating caused by sympathetic stimulation.
- Rapid, weak pulse caused by tachycardia and decreased stroke volume.
- Reduced pulse pressure.
- Rapid, shallow breathing.
- Impaired renal output.
- Muscular weakness.
- Confusion or reduced awareness.

Hypovolemic shock
This results from a fall in circulating blood volume caused by either:
- External fluid loss (e.g., vomiting, diarrhea, hemorrhage).
- Internal fluid loss (e.g., pancreatitis, severe burns, internal bleeding).

Septicemic shock
Septicemic shock is caused by toxins (e.g., endotoxin) released from bacteria during infection. The patient may have warm skin but will have a low blood pressure due to inappropriate vasodilatation. Treatment can include epinephrine and vasoconstrictors. Artificial ventilation is sometimes required for lung involvement if respiratory distress syndrome develops.

Cardiogenic shock
This is caused by an interruption of cardiac function such that the heart is unable to maintain the circulation. It usually has an acute onset, but it may be a result of worsening heart failure. Causes include the following:
- Myocardial infarction.
- Arrhythmia.
- Cardiac tamponade.
- Myocarditis.
- Infective endocarditis.
- Pulmonary embolus.
- Tension pneumothorax.
- Aortic dissection.

Cardiogenic shock should not be treated with epinephrine under any circumstances, because this will exacerbate the cardiac problem.

Anaphylactic shock
This is a type I hypersensitivity reaction, which is an immediate IgE-mediated immune response to an antigen in the body to which the patient is allergic. It leads to circulatory collapse, dyspnea, and even death.

The IgE immune response consists of the activation of basophils and mast cells (basophils are mobile in the blood; mast cells are fixed in tissue). The degranulation of these cells leads to release of histamine and other factors. Prostaglandins, leukotrienes, thromboxane, and platelet activation factors are also synthesized and released. The results are as follows:
- Generalized peripheral vasodilatation, which leads to hypotension.
- Increased vascular permeability reducing plasma volume.
- Bronchial smooth muscle constriction, which leads to dyspnea.

- Oral, laryngeal, and pharyngeal edema.
- Urticaria and flushing.

Death may result from the circulatory collapse.

Treatment consists of immediate administration of epinephrine and infusion of hydrocortisone (a glucocorticoid).

An anaphylactoid reaction produces a similar picture to that just described, but it is caused by the direct effects of a substance on mast cells and basophils (i.e., it is not mediated by IgE). This sometimes occurs with radiopaque contrast media.

Cardiovascular responses to blood loss

A 10% blood loss produces little change in blood pressure. A 20–30% blood loss causes shock, but it is not usually life threatening. A 30–40% blood loss produces severe or irreversible shock (50–70 mmHg fall in blood pressure). Hypotension is an indirect result of blood loss. It is caused by a decreased blood volume, reducing venous return to the heart. Reduced end-diastolic volume reduces the strength of contraction and, therefore, stroke volume.

The body responds in different ways to rectify the loss of pressure and volume. The response is often subdivided into:

- An immediate response occurring within seconds (Fig. 5.1).
- An intermediate response occurring within minutes or hours (Fig. 5.2).
- A long-term response occurring within days or weeks (Fig. 5.3).

Treatment is to prevent further blood loss and volume expansion with intravenous fluids.

 In hemorrhage, the body loses blood. It must attempt to maintain vital perfusion and blood pressure. Then it will try to rectify the loss. The receptors, reflexes, and responses reflect this aim.

Hypertension

In the United States, hypertension is defined as a blood pressure at or above 140/90 mmHg. This value is generally considered to be the point at which the benefits of treatment exceed the risks. Recently, a new category of risk has been defined. Prehypertensive patients are those with a blood pressure in the range of 130–139/80–89 mmHg. This category of patients needs to be carefully monitored

Fig. 5.1 Immediate response to hemorrhage (ADH, antidiuretic hormone; BP, blood pressure; CO, cardiac output; HR, heart rate; SV, stroke volume; TPR, total peripheral resistance).

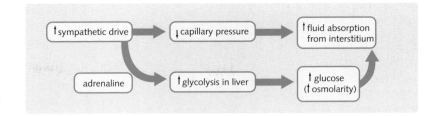

Fig. 5.2 Intermediate response to hemorrhage.

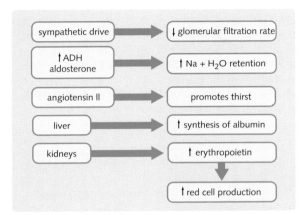

Fig. 5.3 Long-term response to hemorrhage (ADH, antidiuretic hormone).

because they are likely to progress to hypertension. Nonpharmacologic measures should be stressed in this population, with pharmacotherapy considered for patients with a diastolic blood pressure over 85 mmHg. Note that these criteria are determined arbitrarily and that cardiovascular disease risk increases with blood pressure even within the "normal" range. However, based upon these criteria, it is estimated that more than 25% of Americans currently suffer from hypertension, many of them unknowingly, due to the insidious nature of the disease.

Classification

Hypertension is classified according to both underlying cause and clinical progression. Primary (essential) hypertension accounts for 90% of hypertensive patients; the precise etiology is unknown, but it is probably multifactorial. Predisposing factors include:

- Age (blood pressure rises with age).
- Obesity.
- Excessive alcohol intake.
- High salt intake.
- Genetic susceptibility.

Secondary hypertension accounts for the remaining 10% of cases. Here, the hypertension arises as a result of other disease processes:

- Renal disease—chronic glomerulonephritis, chronic pyelonephritis, polycystic renal disease, renal artery stenosis.
- Endocrine disease—Cushing's syndrome, Conn's syndrome, adrenal hyperplasia, pheochromocytoma, acromegaly, corticosteroid therapy.
- Congenital disease—coarctation of the aorta.
- Neurologic disease—raised intracranial pressure, brainstem lesions.
- Pregnancy—pre-eclampsia.

The clinical progression of hypertension can be classified as benign or malignant. Benign hypertension is a stable elevation of blood pressure over a period of many years (usually recognized in patients aged over 40 years). Malignant (accelerated) hypertension is an acute, severe elevation of blood pressure.

Smoking increases cardiovascular risk in all hypertensive patients.

Complications

Hypertension is a major risk factor for:

- Atherosclerosis.
- Intracerebral hemorrhage—also known as cerebrovascular accident (CVA).
- Aortic aneurysm.
- Cardiac failure (which is the cause of death in one third of patients).
- Atrial fibrillation.
- Renal failure.
- Visual disturbance (caused by papilledema and retinal hemorrhages).

Note that initially hypertension is usually asymptomatic, and in essential hypertension no obvious cause can be found. This can affect compliance with therapy, especially if drugs have too many side effects.

The distinction between primary and secondary hypertension is of great clinical significance, since only in the latter case is treatment of the underlying cause possible.

Hypertensive vascular disease

Hypertension not only accelerates atherosclerosis, but it also results in characteristic changes to arterioles and small arteries. All these changes are associated with narrowing of the vessel lumen. Changes in hypertension include:

- In arteries—muscular hypertrophy of the media, reduplication of the external lamina, and intimal thickening.
- In arterioles—hyaline arteriosclerosis (protein deposits in wall).
- In vessels of the brain—microaneurysms (Charcot–Bouchard aneurysms) can occur.

Other changes are associated with, but not restricted to, malignant hypertension. Hyperplastic arteriosclerosis, with reduplication of basement membrane and muscular hypertrophy solely within the intima, can occur in arteries and arterioles.

When these changes are associated with fibrin deposition (also known as fibrinoid changes) and necrosis of the vessel wall, the condition is known as necrotizing arteriolitis. These changes frequently affect the renal arterioles to produce nephrosclerosis, which may impair renal function or exacerbate hypertension through the renin–angiotensin system.

Hypertensive heart disease
Systemic (left-sided) hypertensive heart disease

Criteria for diagnosis of systemic hypertensive heart disease are:

- History of hypertension (>140/90 mmHg).
- Left ventricular hypertrophy (wall thickness measuring >15 mm, weighing >500 g).
- Absence of any other causes of hypertrophy.

In hypertensive heart disease, changes that are initially adaptive lead to cardiac dilatation, congestive heart failure, and even sudden death. The heart adapts with hypertrophy of the left ventricular wall, initially without any change in ventricular volume. Histologically, this is characterized by enlargement of the myocytes and their nuclei (hypertrophy). In the long term, interstitial fibrosis and myocyte atrophy occur, causing ventricular dilatation.

Pulmonary hypertensive heart disease (cor pulmonale)

Pulmonary hypertensive heart disease can be defined as right ventricular hypertrophy (wall thickness measuring >10 mm) as a result of hypertension in the pulmonary circulation caused by a lung disorder.

Pulmonary hypertension can be classified as either:

- Right ventricular hypertrophy and failure (also known as chronic pulmonary hypertension or cor pulmonale).
- Acute pulmonary hypertension (a sudden onset, usually after a large pulmonary embolus).

Right ventricular hypertrophy and failure is a chronic disease of right ventricular pressure load (e.g., pulmonary vasoconstriction in hypoxia caused by high altitude or in chronic obstructive airways disease). Right ventricular dilatation may cause tricuspid regurgitation.

Pulmonary artery hypertension may be caused by heart disease (left ventricular failure, mitral valve disease, cardiac shunts) or lung disease (primary pulmonary hypertension, interstitial fibrosis, pulmonary emboli).

Antihypertensive drugs
Angiotensin-converting enzyme inhibitors

Angiotensin-converting enzyme (ACE) inhibitors (e.g., captopril, enalapril, lisinopril) inhibit the conversion of angiotensin I to angiotensin II by ACE (Fig. 5.4). They also inhibit bradykinin (a vasodilator) breakdown by ACE. They are now becoming a first-line treatment, but they should not be used to treat patients with severe renal artery stenosis.

Some side effects are as follows:

- First-dose hypotension.
- Skin rash.
- Coughing.
- Sore throat.

Risks can be further minimized if the patient takes a once-daily preparation at night when he or she is lying down.

Angiotensin II receptor antagonists

Angiotensin II receptor antagonists (e.g., losartan) inhibit the angiotensin II receptor and prevent the action of angiotensin II (see Fig. 5.4). Unlike the

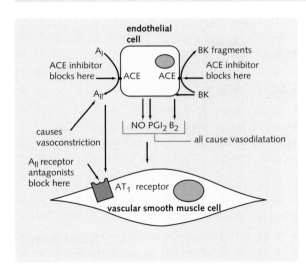

Fig. 5.4 Action of angiotensin-converting enzyme (ACE) inhibitors and angiotensin II (AII) receptor antagonists (AI, angiotensin I, AII, angiotensin II; AT_1, angiotensin II receptor type 1; B_2, activated bradykinin—activated by endothelial cell; BK, bradykinin; NO, nitric oxide; PGI_2, prostacyclin).

ACE inhibitors, they do not affect bradykinin. They are useful when ACE inhibitors have produced an intolerable cough (caused by elevated bradykinin).

Diuretics

Usually a thiazide-type diuretic is used (e.g., hydrochlorothiazide). These drugs inhibit sodium reabsorption in the distal renal tubule, which causes increased salt and water excretion, decreasing blood volume and decreasing blood pressure. Side effects in high doses are:

- Hypokalemia (low K^+) leading to arrhythmia and muscle fatigue.
- Hyperuricemia (high uric acid) causing gout.
- Hyperglycemia (raised blood glucose).
- Increased low-density lipoprotein (LDL) and very-low-density lipoprotein (VLDL), leading to atherosclerosis.

β-blockers

β-blockers are antagonists of β-adrenoceptors. They block sympathetic activity in the heart ($β_1$), peripheral vasculature ($β_2$), and bronchi ($β_2$).

In the heart, this effect decreases heart rate and myocardial contractility. This results in a fall in cardiac output. Renin release from the juxtaglomerular cells is reduced, and there is a

central action, reducing sympathetic drive. These effects combine to lower blood pressure, but only in hypertensive patients.

The effect of β-blockers on the peripheral vasculature leads to a loss of β-mediated vasodilatation, causing an unopposed α-vasoconstriction. This may initially cause an increase in vascular resistance, elevating blood pressure, but in long-term use, the vascular resistance returns to pretreatment levels. However, peripheral blood flow may still be reduced, leading patients to complain of cold extremities.

Some β-blockers can preferentially act on $β_1$-adrenoceptors, being more cardioselective; however, even these drugs have some blocking effect on the $β_2$-adrenoceptor, and they should be given to asthmatic patients with extreme caution.

Types of β-blockers include:

- Propranolol (act on $β_1$, $β_2$).
- Metoprolol, atenolol, bisoprolol (selective $β_1$-blockers).

The main side effects of β-blockers are:

- Bronchoconstriction, leading to worsening asthma or chronic obstructive airways disease.
- Bradycardia.
- Hypoglycemia.
- Fatigue and lethargy.
- Impotence.
- Sleep disturbance, nightmares, and vivid dreams (particularly propranolol).
- Rebound hypertension if stopped suddenly.

 Many drugs of the same type have similar suffixes to their names. For example, most β-blockers end in "-ol" (e.g., propranolol, atenolol, metoprolol). This is useful when identifying the type of an unfamiliar drug.

α-blockers

α-blockers (e.g., prazosin and doxazosin) are antagonists of α-adrenoceptors. They cause postsynaptic block of $α_1$-adrenoceptors, which prevents sympathetic tonic drive and leads to vasodilatation. Therefore, there is a decrease in total peripheral resistance and thus a decrease in blood pressure. Doxazosin is often used for labile (catecholamine-mediated) hypertension.

Side effects of α-blockers are:
- Postural hypotension caused by loss of sympathetic vasoconstriction.
- First-dose phenomenon of rapid hypotension when initially administered.

Other sympatholytics

Adrenergic neuron blockers (e.g., guanethidine) prevent the release of norepinephrine from postganglionic neurons. They are rarely used now because they affect supine blood pressure control and may cause postural hypotension. They may be useful with other therapy in resistant hypertension.

Centrally acting α_2-agonists (e.g., methyldopa, clonidine) decrease central sympathetic drive. Methyldopa enters the neuronal cell, where it is transported into the storage vesicle and metabolized to methyl-norepinephrine, a more selective α_2-receptor agonist. Clonidine enters the CNS and stimulates α_2 receptors without conversion. Stimulation of α_2 receptors serves a "feedback" function on the neuron and suppresses further neurotransmitter release and sympathetic outflow to the periphery. These drugs, primarily methyldopa, are commonly used to treat hypertension associated with pregnancy because they are efficacious and safe. There are insufficient data on most more modern antihypertensive drugs to warrant risking their use.

Calcium antagonists

Calcium antagonists (e.g., verapamil, nifedipine, amlodipine, diltiazem) block voltage-gated calcium channels in myocardium and vascular smooth muscle. This causes a decrease in myocardial contractility and electrical conductance and decreased vascular tone.

Calcium antagonists interfere with the action of various vasoconstrictor agonists (e.g., norepinephrine, angiotensin II, thrombin). All may precipitate heart failure (but this risk is reduced with nifedipine and nifedipine-like drugs, such as amlodipine).

Verapamil decreases cardiac output and heart rate (antiarrhythmic activity), but it should not be used with β-blockers, because it causes hypotension and may lead to asystole. The main side effect of verapamil is constipation.

Nifedipine and amlodipine relax vascular smooth muscle, dilating arteries. The main side effects are headache and ankle edema.

Diltiazem also decreases vascular tone. This is often effective in angina. Its main side effect is bradycardia.

Potassium channel agonists

Potassium channel agonists (e.g., minoxidil and diazoxide) open ATP-dependent K^+ channels. Opening of K^+ channels hyperpolarizes vascular smooth muscle cells, thereby making depolarization harder to achieve. This reduces the stimulation by vasoconstricting agonists on the muscle cells.

Potassium channel agonists are used only in severe hypertension when other methods have failed (diazoxide is used in hypertensive emergencies). They are usually used with a β-blocker and thiazide diuretic to counteract side effects.

Side effects of potassium channel agonists are:
- Increased hair growth (with minoxidil).
- Salt and water retention, leading to edema (use thiazide).
- Reflex sympathetic activation causing tachycardia (use β-blocker).

Sodium nitroprusside

Sodium nitroprusside is an inorganic nitrate with a powerful vasodilator effect. It spontaneously breaks down into nitric oxide (NO), causing vascular smooth muscle relaxation. Sodium nitroprusside should only be used intravenously to control severe hypertensive crises (acute emergency situations). The side effects are excessive hypotension and cyanide toxicity (cyanide is a metabolite, causing tachycardia, metabolic acidosis, and arrhythmia—give sodium nitrite and sodium thiocyanate). Sodium nitroprusside should always be used with a β-blocker to prevent severe reflex tachycardia.

Combinations

ACE inhibitors are being used increasingly as a first-line treatment for hypertension, because they carry a reduced risk of side effects. They can be combined with thiazide treatment, but caution should be used with existing diuretic treatment due to the risk of a collapse in blood pressure in volume-depleted patients. β-blockers have traditionally been used with a thiazide if a thiazide has not been effective alone.

After these options have failed or are contraindicated, calcium antagonists should be tried.

Diuretics may also be used, but verapamil should not be combined with β-blockers.

In severe hypertension where the above therapies have been tried or are contraindicated, the vasodilators, α-blockers, and centrally acting drugs may be used. They may be used in conjunction with an ACE inhibitor, or a thiazide and a β-blocker, although doxazosin is being used more frequently in preference to diuretics and β-blockers because of its vasodilator effect and minimal side effects.

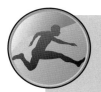

The adverse effects of drugs can usually be divided into types A and B.
- Type A effects are predictable.
- Type B effects are idiosyncratic.

For example, hypotension as a side effect of β-blockers is predictable, because their action is to decrease blood pressure—this is a type A effect. However, skin rashes occur as a hypersensitivity reaction—this is a type B effect.

Special patient populations

Antihypertensive drug choice is especially important in some patient populations and in patients with comorbid conditions. Drug choice in these patients needs to be optimized to produce maximal benefit without exacerbating untoward effects. For example, many African-Americans do not respond well to β-blockers, ACE inhibitors, or ARBs. A more favorable response may be achieved with diuretics or calcium channel blockers. Similarly, older patients often suffer from a special type of hypertension termed "isolated systolic hypertension." This form of hypertension is usually treated with calcium channel blockers or diuretics. Patients suffering from angina pectoris or migraine headaches may be effectively treated with β-blockers, which will also help treat the comorbid condition. ACE inhibitors or ARBs are a good choice in patients with left ventricular dysfunction and in patients suffering from diabetic nephropathy.

Lipids and the cardiovascular system

Lipid transport and metabolism

The insolubility of lipids in plasma means a special transport mechanism is required. This is provided by lipid–protein complexes known as lipoproteins, while the individual proteins are known as apolipoproteins. The apolipoproteins also act as receptors for cell surface proteins, which determine the destination of different lipoproteins. Low-density lipoprotein (LDL) is the main lipoprotein involved in the transport of cholesterol. Fig. 5.5 shows the main transport pathways for lipids from the diet (exogenous) and for lipids from the body's stores (endogenous).

It is thought that lipoprotein A is a prothrombotic lipoprotein that is particularly involved in coronary disease, while high levels of high-density lipoprotein (HDL) are protective. The classification of lipoproteins is outlined in Fig. 5.6.

Hyperlipidemia

Hyperlipidemia (Fig. 5.7) can be classified as hypertriglyceridemia (raised triglycerides—also called triacylglycerides), hypercholesterolemia (raised cholesterol), or hyperlipoproteinemia (raised lipoproteins).

Effects of hyperlipidemia
Atherosclerosis

There is a strong correlation between cholesterol levels and death rates from ischemic vascular disease. There is an even stronger correlation between fibrinogen levels and ischemic vascular disease. It must therefore be remembered that atherosclerosis is a multifactorial disease.

It is thought that LDL damages the arterial wall (or exacerbates wall injury from other causes) by producing oxygen radicals. This may be opposed by the administration of antioxidants (e.g., vitamin E). Atheromatous plaques may develop in this damaged arterial wall.

Atherosclerosis occurs at a young age in some familial hyperlipidemias, but not others.

HDL protects against atherosclerosis.

Acute pancreatitis

Acute pancreatitis can result from hypertriglyceridemia.

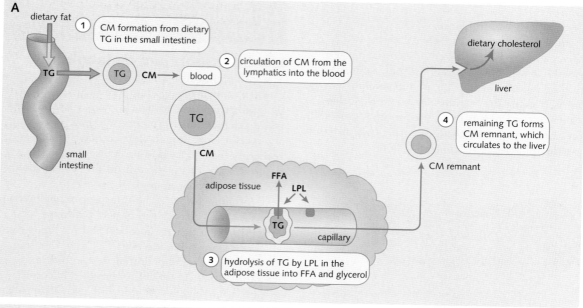

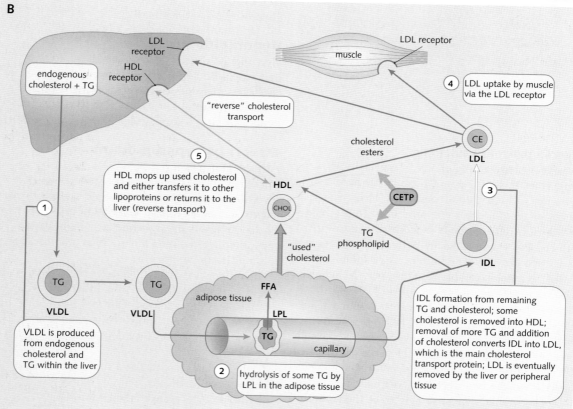

Fig. 5.5 Exogenous (A) and endogenous (B) lipid transport pathways (CE, cholesterol esters; CETP, cholesterol ester transfer protein; CM, chylomicron; FFA, free fatty acid; HDL, high-density lipoprotein; IDL, intermediate-density lipoprotein; LDL, low-density lipoprotein; LPL, lipoprotein lipase; TG, triacylglycerol; VLDL, very low-density lipoprotein).

Classification of lipoproteins		
Particle	**Source**	**Predominantly transports**
Chylomicron (CM)	Gut	Triacylglycerol
Very low-density lipoprotein (VLDL)	Liver	Triacylglycerol
Intermediate-density lipoprotein (IDL)	Catabolism	Cholesterol
Low-density lipoprotein (LDL)	Catabolism	Cholesterol
High-density lipoprotein (HDL)	Catabolism	Cholesterol
Lipoprotein A	Liver, gut	–

Fig. 5.6 Classification of lipoproteins.

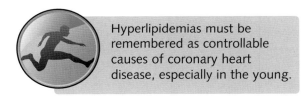

Hyperlipidemias must be remembered as controllable causes of coronary heart disease, especially in the young.

Xanthomas

These are painful deposits of lipids in the skin and in tendons. They are usually diagnostic of hyperlipidemia.

Treatment of hyperlipidemia

Hyperlipidemia can be treated by diet or drugs.

Dietary treatment involves reduction of caloric intake, saturated fats, cholesterol, and alcohol; supplements of omega–3 fats (present in fish oils) may be given to increase HDL levels, which is beneficial.

Indications for drug therapy are:
- High LDL levels, which must be treated if arterial disease is present.
- High triglycerides, which need to be treated only if symptomatic (e.g., causing xanthomas or pancreatitis).
- Low HDL levels.

Drugs used to lower triglyceride levels
Nicotinic acid

Nicotinic acid inhibits VLDL synthesis by the liver, leading to a decrease in intermediate-density lipoprotein (IDL) and LDL. It also increases lipoprotein lipase (LPL) activity.

Nicotinic acid can be used for most types of hyperlipidemia, usually in conjunction with a resin (see below). Its main side effects are rashes, nausea, abnormal liver function, and a prostaglandin-mediated cutaneous reaction. Its use has declined in favor of a statin (e.g., simvastatin).

Fibrates

Gemfibrozil reduces lipolysis of triglycerides in adipose tissue, leading to decreased hepatic production of VLDL. Bezafibrate increases LPL activity, which leads to decreased VLDL and decreased triglycerides, but it may increase LDL.

Fibrates are used mainly in familial type III hyperlipidemia. Gemfibrozil is the better drug, because it does not increase LDL. The main side effects include nausea, abdominal discomfort, and flu-like symptoms.

Drugs used to lower cholesterol
Bile acid-binding resins (e.g., colestipol and cholestyramine)

Colestipol and cholestyramine inhibit reabsorption of cholesterol in the gut. They bind to bile salts in the gut and stop their reabsorption. This leads to increased excretion and decreased absorption of cholesterol. To compensate, the liver increases cholesterol conversion into bile salts and also increases LDL receptors. This removes LDL cholesterol from circulation. They can aggravate hypertriglyceridemia.

Statins (e.g., simvastatin and pravastatin)

Simvastatin and pravastatin are β-hydroxy-β-methylglutaryl coenzyme A (HMG CoA) reductase inhibitors. The liver compensates for the decreased cholesterol synthesis by increasing LDL receptors, which decrease plasma levels of LDL cholesterol. They are used to treat most hypercholesterolemias, and they are very effective if used in conjunction with a resin (up to 50% reduction in cholesterol levels). They are currently the only lipid-lowering treatment for which there is good evidence for reduced mortality.

Classification of hyperlipidemias					
Condition	Elevated lipoprotein	Elevated lipid	Biochemical defect	Drug therapy	Prevalence
Single gene defect					
Familial lipoprotein lipase (LPL) deficiency (type I)	CMs	Triacylglyceride	Low or absent LPL activity	Diet alone	Rare
Familial hypercholesterolemia (type IIa)	LDL	Cholesterol	Deficiency of LDL receptors (none in homozygotic	Statin, resin	Common
Familial combined hyperlipidemia (type IIb)	VLDL, LDL	Triacylglyceride, cholesterol	Overproduction of apo-B	Fibrate	Common
Familial hyperlipoproteinemia (type III)	CM remnants, IDL	Triacylglyceride, cholesterol	Abnormal apo-E	Fibrate	Rare
Familial hypertriglyceridemia (type IV)	VLDL	Triacylglyceride	Overproduction of VLDL by the liver	Fibrate	Common
Familial hypertriglyceridemia (type V)	VLDL, CMs	Triacylglyceride, cholesterol	Overproduction of VLDL by the liver	Fibrate	Rare
Multifactorial					
Hypertriglyceridemia	VLDL	Triacylglyceride	Unknown	Fibrate	Common
Hypercholesterolemia	LDL	Cholesterol	Unknown	Statin, resin	Common

Fig. 5.7 Classification of hyperlipidemias. Familial, heritable abnormalities of lipid metabolism are classified according to Fredrickson type (types I–V) on the underlying genetic mutations. Hyperlipidemia may also be multifactorial or idiopathic, without a currently identified or discrete genetic basis. These are clinically the most common in older patients (CM, chylomicron; IDL, intermediate-density lipoprotein; LDL, low-density lipoprotein; VLDL, very low-density lipoprotein).

The main side effects include reversible myositis and disturbed liver function tests.

Probucol

Probucol causes a 10% reduction in LDL cholesterol, but it also lowers HDL and remains in the body for months. It has some antioxidant activity, which may reduce atherosclerosis formation.

Arteriosclerosis and atherosclerosis

Definitions and concepts

Arteriosclerosis is a term used to describe hardening and thickening of arteries. This reduces their elastic properties. Atherosclerosis is one of the processes that produces arteriosclerosis. It involves the formation of atheroma, which is an accumulation of lipid plaques within the walls of a vessel. Arteriosclerosis of small arteries and arterioles is termed "arteriolosclerosis" and is mainly caused by hypertension.

There are two main types of arteriosclerosis:
- Atherosclerosis.
- Arteriolosclerosis.

Consequences of arteriosclerosis

Arteriosclerosis results in a reduced arterial lumen with a consequent loss in perfusion. Furthermore, due to the loss of elasticity, rupture is more likely. There is also a predisposition to thrombus formation.

Atherosclerosis

It has been said that every adult in the Western world has some degree of atheroma in his or her arteries. Atherosclerosis and its complications are the main cause of mortality (more than 50%) in the Western world. The incidence of atherosclerosis is rising in the United States.

Risk factors

Risk factors for atherosclerosis include constitutional factors such as:

- Age. Increased age increases the number and severity of lesions.
- Male sex. Men are affected to a much greater extent than women, until menopause, when the incidence in women increases; but men continue to be predominantly affected. This is thought to be because of the protective effect of estrogens.
- Genetic predisposition.

Strong risk factors for atherosclerosis are:

- Smoking.
- Hypertension.
- Diabetes mellitus (see p. 88).
- Hyperlipidemia. It is directly related to levels of cholesterol and LDL. HDL levels are protective.
- Hyperfibrinogenemia.
- Hyperhomocysteinemia.

Other factors involved in the development of atherosclerosis are:

- Exercise—decreases the incidence of coronary heart disease; however, whether it prevents atheroma formation is unclear.
- Obesity—increases mortality, but this may only be a reflection of diet and lipid profile.
- Diet—decreased saturated fat intake has a beneficial effect, as may antioxidants (e.g., vitamin E in red wine).
- Stress and personality—certain highly stressed and type A personalities may have an increased tendency to atherosclerosis and coronary heart disease, but these data are inconclusive.

Pathogenesis

Atherosclerosis generally affects medium to large arteries. It is characterized by lipid deposition in the intima, with smooth muscle and matrix proliferation combining to produce a fibrous plaque that protrudes into the lumen (Fig. 5.8). The lesions tend to be focal, patchy, and do not involve the whole circumference of the vessel.

Certain stages (see Fig. 5.8) are postulated to occur in atheroma formation, according to the "response to injury" hypothesis.

Other theories of pathogenesis include:

- Neoplasia. An abnormal proliferation of smooth muscle occurs, caused by some as yet unidentified factor that produces uncontrolled growth.
- Prostaglandins. The balance between prostacyclin and thromboxane has an influence on thrombus formation, and because fibrin and platelets are important components of atheromatous lesions, this must have a strong influence on pathogenesis.
- Thrombosis is the primary event that builds up in layers and organizes to form atheromatous plaques.

Atherosclerosis is primarily an inflammatory process, and it is asymptomatic until it produces:

- Narrowing of the lumen—sufficient narrowing of the vessel produces symptoms of ischemia (e.g., intermittent claudication, angina, or gangrene).
- Sudden occlusion—caused by plaque rupture followed by thrombosis (e.g., in myocardial infarction).
- Emboli—these may have an impact in other vessels.
- Aneurysms—resulting from wall weakening.

There is a high mortality associated with the formation of atheromatous plaques. A knowledge of how an atheroma is thought to occur is therefore helpful on the national boards.

Treatment

The majority of research has looked at ways of reducing ischemic heart disease by treating risk factors; it is not known what effect this has on the progress of atherosclerosis, but indirectly the following treatments have been used:

- Dietary control (reduced fat and sugar intake; increased amounts of fresh fruit and vegetables).
- Regular exercise and change in lifestyle (decrease stress).
- Stopping smoking.
- Cholesterol-lowering drugs (e.g., statins).

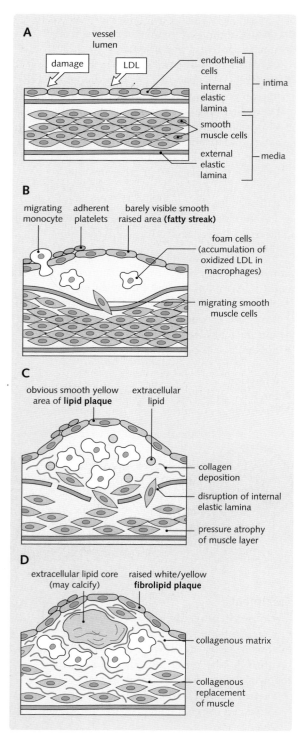

A
- vessel lumen
- damage
- LDL
- endothelial cells
- internal elastic lamina
- intima
- smooth muscle cells
- external elastic lamina
- media

B
- migrating monocyte
- adherent platelets
- barely visible smooth raised area (**fatty streak**)
- foam cells (accumulation of oxidized LDL in macrophages)
- migrating smooth muscle cells

C
- obvious smooth yellow area of **lipid plaque**
- extracellular lipid
- collagen deposition
- disruption of internal elastic lamina
- pressure atrophy of muscle layer

D
- extracellular lipid core (may calcify)
- raised white/yellow **fibrolipid plaque**
- collagenous matrix
- collagenous replacement of muscle

Fig. 5.8 Stages in the formation of an atheromatous plaque. A. Damage to the endothelium. Chronic or repeated endothelial cell (EC) injury occurs, leading to metabolic dysfunction and structural changes. ECs have a

Mönckeberg's medial calcific sclerosis

Mönckeberg's medial calcific sclerosis is a specific type of arteriosclerosis. It is an idiopathic, degenerative disease of the elderly (more than 50 years old) characterized by focal calcifications in the media of small- and medium-sized arteries.

The femoral, tibial, radial, and ulnar arteries are predominantly involved. There is little or no inflammation, and usually the calcifications do not cause either obstructions or symptoms. There is an increase in pulse pressure (systolic hypertension) caused by loss of elasticity in the arteries.

Effects of diabetes mellitus on vessels

Diabetes mellitus causes a range of serious vascular complications, the severity of which is directly related to blood glucose levels. Intensive control of blood glucose (monitored long term by levels of glycosylated hemoglobin, HbA_{1c}) and treatment with ACE inhibitors can minimize these risks. Complications include:

- Microangiopathy.
- Hyaline arteriosclerosis.
- Atherosclerosis.

major role in actively preventing thrombus formation. Damage activates EC, upregulating inflammatory adhesion molecules (e.g., ICAM–1) and promoting monocyte and platelet adhesion. Injury also increases permeability to lipids and low-density lipoprotein (LDL), allowing movement into the intima. B. Formation of a fatty streak. Monocytes adhere to the endothelium, migrate into the intima, and become macrophages. There they take up the LDL and become foam cells, because they cannot degrade lipids. Local oxidation of LDL aids uptake by, and is chemotactic for, macrophages. Platelets adhere to activated endothelial cells or areas of denuded matrix. Activated platelets, activated EC, and macrophages release platelet-derived growth factor (PDGF) and induce smooth muscle migration into the intima. C. Development of lipid plaque. Smooth muscle proliferation and an increase in extracellular matrix occur in the intima. Smooth muscle cells also take up LDL and form foam cells. Greater macrophage infiltration takes place. Lipid may also be released free into the intima. Macrophages contribute many other factors (e.g., superoxide, proteases) that increase the damage. D. Complicated plaques. As the lesion develops, pressure causes the media to atrophy and the muscle to be replaced by collagen. A fibrous cap of collagen forms on top. There is increased free lipid in the intima. The endothelium becomes fragile and ulcerates, leading to further platelet aggregation and thrombus formation.

muscle. They mainly cause vasodilatation, and they are used in both angina of effort and vasospastic angina:

- Angina of effort. Calcium channel blockers decrease total peripheral resistance, lessening the demand on the heart.
- Vasospastic angina. These drugs cause relaxation of spasm.

Side effects of calcium channel blockers are:

- Headache and facial flushing.
- Constipation.
- Reflex tachycardia.
- Edema.

Verapamil should not be combined with β-blockers, while nifedipine may be beneficially combined with β-blockers to minimize reflex tachycardia.

Antiplatelet Therapy

Antiplatelet therapy aimed at reducing the risk of platelet aggregation and subsequent thrombotic episodes should be a part of the treatment regimen in all patients suffering from ischemic heart disease. For most patients, this can be accomplished with aspirin, which has the added benefit of an anti-inflammatory action that may stabilize atheromatous plaques. For patients in whom aspirin is contraindicated, agents such as clodiprogel should be strongly considered.

β-blockers

These drugs block sympathetic stimulation of the heart, leading to:

- Decreased force and, therefore, decreased oxygen demand.
- Decreased rate and, therefore, decreased oxygen demand and also increased time for oxygen supply.

They are used in angina of effort, but not in vasospastic angina, because they have no dilatory effect. They should not be used to treat patients with asthma, peripheral arterial disease, or bradyarrhythmias.

The mechanism and treatment of angina are frequently questions on the national boards.

Myocardial infarction

Myocardial infarction is classified as:

- Subendocardial myocardial infarction—affecting the innermost region of the myocardium.
- Transmural myocardial infarction—affecting the full thickness of one segment of the myocardium.

Myocardial infarction occurs when an area of muscle of the heart dies (i.e., undergoes necrosis). It is caused by a reduction or blockage in the coronary blood supply, and it is usually precipitated by thrombosis or hemorrhage in an atherosclerotic area of a coronary artery. There are many complications, including arrhythmias, heart failure, and even sudden death.

Myocardial infarctions can be classified into two broad categories, subendocardial and transmural. It was previously thought that transmural infarctions initially elevated the ST-segment, followed by the appearance of Q waves, while subendocardial infarctions initially depressed the Q wave and did not lead to the development of Q waves. More recent evidence does not support such a tight correlation between ECG abnormalities and pathologic findings; however, the distinction is still useful, because patients suffering from non-Q wave infarctions have a lower rate of hospital mortality. Long-term follow-up, however, demonstrates that these patients have a high rate of reinfarction and mortality, probably because they often suffer from multivessel disease and are subject to recurrent ischemia. Thus, aggressive treatment of these patients is warranted.

Subendocardial myocardial infarction

This is an infarction of the subendocardial layer of the myocardium. Diffuse atherosclerosis is usually present in all three main arteries. The infarction is caused by:

- Increased demand.
- Decreased blood supply.
- Hypotension.
- Vasospasm.

It may or may not involve a superimposed thrombosis. Injury is less severe than that of transmural infarcts and can be diffuse or regional.

Transmural myocardial infarction

A transmural infarction affects the full thickness of the myocardium. It usually involves an occlusion of a major coronary artery, causing ischemia to a specific region of the heart. Transmural myocardial infarction may be caused by:

- An acute plaque change (ulceration, fissuring, or hemorrhage) leading to thrombosis.
- Platelet aggregation.
- Vasospasm (rarely).

If sufficient collateral blood flow is present, complete occlusion of a vessel may not lead to an infarction, because the collateral flow may adequately perfuse the tissue.

Nearly all infarcts affect the left ventricle; 15% involve both ventricles, and 3% involve just the right ventricle. The arteries commonly infarcted are:

- Left anterior descending artery (50%)—affecting the left ventricular anterior wall and interventricular septum.
- Right coronary artery (30%)—affecting the left ventricular inferior and posterior walls and right ventricle.
- Left circumflex artery (20%)—affecting the left ventricular lateral wall.

From the onset of ischemia, it takes only 20–40 minutes until irreversible injury starts to occur. Reperfusion (the return of flow) caused by thrombolysis (spontaneous or drug induced) can lessen the extent of damage; however, reperfused myocytes may not function to the same level for a few days. A characteristic series of events occurs (Fig. 5.11).

Sudden death occurs in 25% of patients, usually as a result of an arrhythmia; 90% of survivors develop acute or chronic complications. Acute complications include:

- Arrhythmias.
- Heart failure.
- Cardiogenic shock.
- Ventricular rupture.
- Papillary muscle infarction, leading to mitral valve incompetence.
- Mural thrombosis, leading to pulmonary or peripheral thromboembolism.
- Pericarditis.

Chronic complications include:
- Ventricular aneurysm and thrombosis.
- Recurrent infarction.
- Arrhythmias.
- Chronic heart failure.

Mortality is 35% in the first year, and 10% every year thereafter.

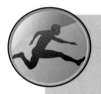 The time course of microscopic and macroscopic changes in the myocardium following an MI is a popular topic for board questions. Make sure you review them carefully.

Events occurring after myocardial infarction		
Time after myocardial infarction	**Macroscopic events**	**Microscopic events**
6–12 h	Normal	Edema
12–18 h	Normal	Neutrophils appear
18–24 h	Pale or cyanotic	Myocyte necrosis
1–3 days	Hyperemic border	Inflammation
3–7 days	Yellow, sharply defined lesion that softens	Dead cells disintegrate and are mopped up by macrophages
7–10 days	Hemorrhagic edge	Granulation tissue replaces dead tissue
12 days	Scar formation	Dense fibrous tissue

Fig. 5.11 Time line of events occurring after infarction.

Treatment
Fibrinolytic drugs
Thrombolytic (fibrinolytic) therapy is used to break down the thrombi that cause a myocardial infarction. If given within 3 hours, it probably allows reperfusion in about half the affected arteries.

Thrombolytics include:
- Streptokinase—binds and activates plasminogen to form plasmin, causing fibrinolysis. Plasmin also lyses fibrinogen and prothrombin (anticoagulant effect). Streptokinase must be used cautiously, because it can cause anaphylactic reactions.
- Anistreplase (APSAC)—is metabolized to streptokinase.
- (Recombinant) tissue plasminogen activator—(r)tPA—may be used when patients are suspected to be sensitive to streptokinase, because it does

not cause any allergic anaphylactic reactions. It is increasingly used in large anterior infarctions in accordance with the results of the Global Utilization of Streptokinase and Tissue Plasminogen Activator for Occluded Coronary Arteries (GUSTO) trials (a series of global studies of cardiovascular disease treatments). It must be given with heparin.

Several trials have shown that all three fibrinolytic drugs are generally equally effective in the treatment of acute myocardial infarction, although the GUSTO trials have shown that tPA may be more beneficial in high-risk patients, albeit with a higher incidence of stroke. Side effects include:
- Nausea and vomiting.
- Bleeding (may result in strokes).

Nonsteroidal anti-inflammatory drugs (NSAIDs)

Aspirin is an NSAID that irreversibly inhibits the cyclooxygenase enzyme. It has been shown to be beneficial in an acute myocardial infarction (with streptokinase) and in preventing myocardial infarction and stroke.

Aspirin's beneficial effects in thromboembolic disease are thought to be caused by decreased synthesis of thromboxane A_2 ($Tx-A_2$) by platelets. $Tx-A_2$ is a strong inducer of platelet aggregation. Its action is antagonized by prostacyclin (PGI_2) from endothelial cells. PGI_2 synthesis is also blocked by aspirin, but the endothelial cell is able to produce more cyclooxygenase enzyme (this cannot occur in platelets because they have no nucleus). The overall action, therefore, is to inhibit platelet aggregation.

Side effects include the following:
- Bronchospasm.
- Gastrointestinal hemorrhage.

Sudden cardiac death

Sudden cardiac death is unexpected death from a cardiac cause within 1 hour of onset of symptoms. There is usually plaque disruption, but ultimately death is caused by a fatal arrhythmia (asystole or ventricular fibrillation) due to scarring of the conduction system, acute ischemic injury, or electrolyte imbalance.

Heart failure

Definition

Heart failure (cardiac failure) is said to have occurred when the heart is no longer able to maintain circulation to the tissues adequately enough to support normal metabolism.

Conditions

Conditions that lead to heart failure can be broadly divided into:
- Those that damage cardiac muscle (e.g., ischemic heart disease, cardiomyopathies).
- Those that demand extra work of the heart (e.g., systemic hypertension, valvular heart disease).

Symptoms and signs

Symptoms and signs of heart failure include:
- Muscle fatigue.
- Reduced exercise tolerance.
- Tachycardia.
- Dyspnea, possibly caused by increased fluid in the lungs.
- Orthopnea (shortness of breath while lying flat).
- Paroxysmal nocturnal dyspnea (sudden shortness of breath while sleeping).
- Hemoptysis caused by increased venous pressure, leading to alveolar hemorrhage.
- Elevated jugular venous pressure (due to venous congestion).
- Hepatomegaly (due to venous congestion).
- Edema (due to venous congestion).
- Proteinuria caused by prerenal renal failure.

 Remember, "heart failure" is *not* a diagnosis. You must *always* identify the underlying pathology that is responsible.

Compensatory mechanisms

There is a decrease in contractility of the affected heart muscle in chronic heart failure. This shifts the Starling curve to the right and downward and reduces the force of contraction for a given filling pressure (Fig. 5.12). The body attempts to compensate by increasing filling pressure (Fig. 5.13).

This is achieved by:
- Catecholamine release secondary to increased sympathetic nerve activity, increasing heart rate and force.
- Peripheral vasoconstriction/venoconstriction, which will increase filling pressure but also total peripheral resistance (this increases the demand on the heart).
- Renal retention of Na^+ and water to increase blood volume and filling pressure, also causing edema.

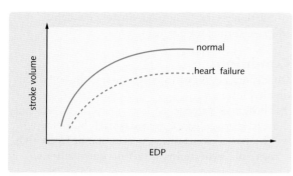

Fig. 5.12 The Starling curve in heart failure. Reduced contractility reduces stroke volume for a given filling pressure (EDP, end-diastolic pressure).

These responses only confer a limited benefit. Increased cardiac filling initially increases cardiac output through Starling's law, but prolonged excessive cardiac filling causes excessive dilatation. This leads to ineffective contraction and causes the heart to enlarge (hypertrophy) and eventually fail. According to Laplace's law, dilatation of the heart requires the myocytes to increase the tension in the wall to sustain the same pressure. This increases oxygen demand and predisposes the myocardium to ischemia. Dilatation may also ultimately lead to valvular incompetence. A key aim for treatment, therefore, is to reduce the load on the failing heart (e.g., by venodilation),

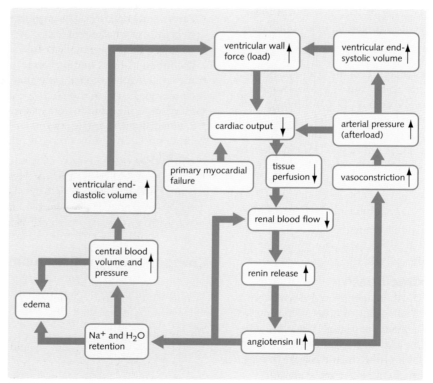

Fig. 5.13 The series of changes in heart failure is initiated by myocardial changes, which impair the efficiency of the heart. Causes include infarction, cardiomyopathy, and chronic hypertension. In the normal heart, an increased end-diastolic or systolic volume leads to greater cardiac output by Starling's law, but in a heart with impaired contractility, there is little further reserve. Dilatation of the ventricles further impairs the efficiency of the heart by Laplace's law, requiring greater effort to maintain output. Compensatory changes include sympathetic activation to increase contractility and to raise blood pressure to maintain tissue perfusion, but chronic stimulation leads to an impaired adrenergic response. The renin-angiotensin system is also activated, leading to fluid retention and raised blood pressure. Attempts to raise the systemic blood pressure place further load on an already weakened heart, creating a destructive cycle. Therapy is aimed at controlling these compensatory mechanisms to unload the heart and prevent excessive dilatation.

although this carries a risk of precipitating cardiogenic shock.

Increased catecholamine release (i.e., increased sympathetic drive) results in increased epinephrine and norepinephrine secretion to increase the force and rate of contraction. As the condition worsens, there is an eventual downregulation of β-adrenoceptors reducing this effect.

Treatment of heart failure
Angiotensin-converting enzyme inhibitors
ACE inhibitors (e.g., enalapril, lisinopril, and captopril).
- Block production of angiotensin II and, therefore, aldosterone.
- Prevent the breakdown of bradykinin.
- Prolong life in heart failure.

ACE inhibitors produce vasodilatation/venodilatation, thereby decreasing load and edema. (ACE inhibitors are also used in hypertension.)

β-blockers
The sympatholytic effects of β-blockers have been shown to be beneficial in the long-term management of heart failure. Their action slows the heart, thereby increasing filling time while allowing β-receptor sensitivity to recover. However, they should not be used to treat acute heart failure. Side effects and contraindications have been described previously.

Diuretics
Diuretics increase salt and water excretion, therefore decreasing circulatory volume. This decreases preload and edema. They are classified as:
- Thiazides.
- Loop diuretics.
- Potassium-sparing diuretics.

Thiazides are used in mild cardiac failure and hypertension; loop diuretics are used in moderate and severe heart failure; potassium-sparing diuretics are sometimes used in conjunction with other diuretics to prevent hypokalemia.

Diuretics are often used in combination with an ACE inhibitor.

Thiazides
Thiazides (e.g., chlorothiazide, bendrofluazide, metolazone) prevent Na^+ and Cl^- reabsorption in the distal tubule. Side effects are:

- Hypokalemia.
- Hyperuricemia.
- Hyperlipidemia.
- Hyperglycemia.
- Potential allergic reactions.

Loop diuretics
Loop diuretics (e.g., furosemide and bumetanide) inhibit NaCl reabsorption in the loop of Henle. They cause more potent diuresis than other diuretics, and they can be used in patients with reduced renal function. Side effects are:
- Hypokalemia.
- Ototoxicity.
- Hyperuricemia.
- Hypomagnesemia.
- Potential allergic reactions.

Potassium-sparing diuretics
Potassium-sparing diuretics (e.g., spironolactone and amiloride) antagonize the effect of aldosterone (spironolactone) or may block Na^+ channels in the distal tubule. The effect is to prevent Na^+ reabsorption and K^+ excretion. Spironolactone has been shown to prolong life in heart failure. The main side effect is hyperkalemia, a major risk when combined with ACE inhibitors.

Inotropic drugs
Inotropic drugs increase the contractility of the myocardium. Their principal role should be restricted to the management of acute heart failure, because they are associated with increased mortality with long-term use.

They can be classified as:
- Cardiac glycosides.
- $β_1$-sympathomimetics.
- Phosphodiesterase inhibitors.

Cardiac glycosides
Cardiac glycosides (e.g., digoxin and ouabain) inhibit the sodium pump, which leads to a rise in intracellular Ca^{2+} in many cells. This:
- Increases the force of contraction via actions on the myocardium.
- Reduces sympathetic outflow via actions on arterial baroreceptors.
- Promotes fluid excretion via actions on the kidney.

They also have a central effect to increase vagal activity, which slows the heart rate.

The side effects of cardiac glycosides include:
- Anorexia.
- Nausea and vomiting.
- Diarrhea.
- Confusion.
- Arrhythmia in toxic doses.

Cardiac glycosides are contraindicated in hypokalemia because of potentiation of their action, and they should be combined with thiazides and loop diuretics with caution.

β_1-sympathomimetics
The β_1-sympathomimetics dobutamine and dopamine increase the force of contraction. Dopamine also increases renal blood flow in low doses. Side effects are tachycardia and hypertension in overdose.

Phosphodiesterase inhibitors (milrinone)
Milrinone inhibits phosphodiesterase, which is the enzyme that breaks down cyclic adenosine monophosphate (cAMP) into 5'-AMP. Inhibition causes a rise in intracellular cAMP and, therefore, Ca^{2+}. This means there is an increase in contractility. Milrinone is also a vasodilator. It is used in severe heart failure that is unresponsive to other therapy.

Arrhythmia

Definitions and classification
An arrhythmia is any deviation from the heart's normal sinus rhythm. Descriptions of arrhythmias are outlined below. Arrhythmias are usually classified clinically as supraventricular or ventricular.
- Supraventricular—originating in the atrium or atrioventricular node.
- Ventricular—originating in the ventricle.

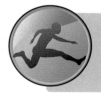 Sinus rhythms are termed "sinus" because they arise from the sinus node and follow the normal electrical path.

Altered sinus rhythms
Sinus tachycardia and sinus bradycardia are produced by autonomic nervous activity. It usually takes several beats to produce a new steady state.

Tachycardia (>100 beats/min in adults) usually results from:
- Exercise.
- Emotion.
- Fever.
- Sinus tachycardia will show normal P waves, with a stable P–R interval within normal limits.

Bradycardia (<60 beats/min) commonly occurs in:
- Athletes.
- Patients with raised intracranial pressure.

Sinus arrhythmia generally manifests in the young as a change in rhythm with respiration. The heart rate increases with inspiration and decreases with expiration.

Extrasystole (ectopic beats)
Extrasystole occurs when an abnormal beat is generated in an area of myocardium before the next sinus beat. The impulse that is generated goes on to contract the ventricle. Atrial extrasystole or ventricular extrasystole may occur, depending upon the area of origin. Usually, there is a gap before the next normal sinus beat; this is termed the "compensatory phase."

Atrial (supraventricular) tachycardia and atrial flutter
Atrial tachycardia and atrial flutter are caused by an abnormal focus in the atrium or by an abnormal conduction pathway causing re-entry that results in atrial contraction at a rapid rate. It may also be caused by ectopic or junctional beats that may arise from the myocardium surrounding the atrioventricular node, or the tissue forming the "junctional area," which connects the atrioventricular node to the ventricular conduction system. Ectopic beats or abnormal conduction (e.g., Wolff-Parkinson-White syndrome, ischemia) within this area may produce an atrioventricular re-entry tachycardia. P waves may be inverted on an ECG, but they may still cause atrial or ventricular contraction.

In atrial flutter, the rate is usually around 300 beats/min, but not all atrial impulses are conducted to the ventricle. Often, the ratio of atrial to ventricular beats (coupling ratio) is 2:1 or 3:1.

Supraventricular tachycardia is characterized by a heart rate between 140 and 220 beats/min, with narrow QRS complexes.

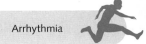

Atrial fibrillation

There is no coordinated atrial activity in atrial fibrillation. A rippling effect of the muscle occurs, which does not contribute to ventricular filling. Ventricular activity is affected, producing a characteristic "irregularly irregular" pulse. It is commonly caused by mitral valve disease, ischemic heart disease, or thyrotoxicosis.

Wolff-Parkinson-White syndrome

In Wolff-Parkinson-White syndrome, there is an extra conduction pathway (the bundle of Kent) between the atria and ventricles. This results in rapid conduction, which can lead to tachycardia or atrial fibrillation.

Heart block (atrioventricular block)

This is an interruption of the normal conduction through the atrioventricular conduction tissue. It may be classified as first-, second-, or third-degree block.

First-degree heart block

In first-degree heart block, all atrial impulses reach the ventricle, but conduction through the atrioventricular tissue takes longer than normal (P–R interval on an electrocardiogram is >0.2 seconds).

Second-degree heart block

In second-degree heart block, some atrial impulses fail to reach the ventricles, but others do (not all P waves are followed by QRS complexes).

Third-degree (complete) heart block

In third-degree heart block, the atria and ventricles beat independently of each other. The ventricular rate is usually about 20–40 beats/min (P waves and QRS complexes have no fixed relationship).

Wenckebach heart block

In Wenckebach heart block, the degree of block increases over a few beats (P–R interval increases over three or four beats, followed by an isolated P wave). Thus, a Wenckebach heart block would be classified as a second-degree heart block.

Ventricular tachycardia

Ventricular tachycardia occurs when impulses originate from an ectopic focus within the ventricles. It is characterized by broad QRS complexes (i.e., duration >120 msec) on an ECG at a rate of >120 beats/min. It is often a precursor to ventricular fibrillation.

Ventricular fibrillation

Ventricular fibrillation is an irregular, uncoordinated rippling contraction of the ventricle. There is no effective cardiac output, leading to rapid loss of consciousness. Death results unless effective treatment is initiated immediately.

Mechanism of arrhythmia

Arrhythmias are caused by a combination of abnormal impulse generation (either an abnormal sinus rhythm or an ectopic pacemaker) or abnormal impulse conduction (re-entry, heart block). A more detailed account of arrhythmia is given in Chapter 8.

Antiarrhythmic drugs

The aims of drug treatment are:
- To decrease cell excitability.
- To increase the refractory period.
- To slow conduction or block conduction if already slow.

The Vaughan-Williams classification system is used for antiarrhythmic drugs; it is based on their actions. It has some limitations because of drugs with multiple actions, but it still serves a useful purpose.

Class I: sodium channel blockers

These drugs can be subdivided into class IA (e.g., quinidine, procainamide, and disopyramide), class IB (e.g., lidocaine, mexiletine, and tocainide), and class IC (e.g., flecainide). They block sodium channels during the open (classes IA and IC) or refractory (class IB) state. They are all "use-dependent" blockers, affecting only active channels.

Class IA: quinidine, procainamide, disopyramide

Class IA drugs prolong the action potential by:
- Increasing the threshold for spontaneous depolarization.
- Slowing the fast upstroke.
- Prolonging the refractory period.

These drugs are used for supraventricular and ventricular arrhythmias. Side effects include:
- Nausea and vomiting.
- Anticholinergic effects—dry mouth, blurred vision, and urinary retention; increased AV nodal conduction.
- Hypotension (disopyramide).
- Precipitation of systemic lupus erythematosus (procainamide).

Quinidine and procainamide should be used with caution due to risks of more severe side effects.

Class IB: lidocaine, mexiletine, tocainide

Class IB drugs bind preferentially to refractory Na^+ channels and therefore act preferentially on ischemic myocardium. They shorten the action potential by:
- Slowing the fast upstroke.
- Increasing the refractory period.

They are used for ventricular arrhythmias, especially after a myocardial infarction. Side effects include:
- Convulsions.
- Nausea and vomiting.

Class IC: flecainide

Class IC drugs have little effect on action potential, but they slow upstroke and conduction speed; there is little change in refractory period. They are used in supraventricular and ventricular arrhythmias. Side effects include:
- Further arrhythmias.
- Dizziness.

Class II: β-adrenergic blockers

Class II drugs (e.g., propranolol and atenolol) block the increase in pacemaker activity that is produced by sympathetic stimulation of β-adrenoceptors. They also slow conduction.

Beta-blockers may be used for ectopic beats, atrial fibrillation, and atrial tachycardia. They are indicated when circulating catecholamines are too high (e.g., after a myocardial infarction and thyrotoxicosis). Side effects include:
- Fatigue.
- Provocation of asthma.

Some drugs (such as sotalol and bretylium) have both class II and III actions.

Class III: potassium channel blockers

Class III drugs (e.g., amiodarone) block K^+ channels, slowing repolarization and leading to a prolonged action potential and refractory period.

Class III drugs are used in supraventricular and ventricular arrhythmias. Side effects of amiodarone include:
- Photosensitivity (turn blue in sun).
- Liver damage.
- Thyroid disorders.

- Neuropathy.
- Pulmonary fibrosis.
- Visual field disturbances.

Amiodarone also has class IA and II effects.

Class IV: calcium channel blockers

Class IV drugs (e.g., verapamil) block calcium channels, thereby decreasing spontaneous activity and conduction at sinoatrial and atrioventricular nodes.

Class IV drugs are used for supraventricular arrhythmias only. Side effects of verapamil are:
- Precipitation of cardiac failure.
- Atrioventricular block.
- Constipation.

Other drugs not in this classification

These include:
- Digitalis (digoxin)—used for supraventricular arrhythmias, especially atrial fibrillation. It has a central effect, stimulating the vagus, causing slowed atrioventricular nodal conduction. This slows the ventricular beat.
- Adenosine—used to terminate supraventricular tachycardias.
- Calcium chloride—used for broad-complex tachycardia.
- Magnesium chloride—used for ventricular fibrillation and to treat digoxin excess.
- Atropine—used to treat bradycardia. It acts by blocking parasympathetic effects on the heart.
- Epinephrine—used in cardiac arrest.
- Isoproterenol—used in the treatment of heart block while awaiting pacing.

Sicilian Gambit classification

In 1991, a group of basic and clinical investigators devised a new classification for antiarrhythmic drugs. Antiarrhythmic drugs fit awkwardly into the Vaughan-Williams classification because of their mixed actions. This new classification provides the best information available on the current antiarrhythmic drugs based on their individual actions. This classification has taken over for the Vaughan-Williams classification but has not yet been universally accepted. A spreadsheet of the actions of current medication has been published (Fig. 5.14).

Drug	Channels						Receptors				Pumps	Clinical effects			Clinical effects		
	Na			Ca	K	I_f	α	β	M₂	A₁	Na⁺/K⁺ ATPase	left ven-tricular function	sinus rate	extra-cardiac	PR interval	QRS width	QT interval
	fast	med	slow														
Lidocaine	□											→	→	▦			↓
Mexiletine	□											→	→	▦			↓
Procainamide		⊘			□							↓	→	■	↑	↑	↑
Disopyramide		⊘			□				□			↓	→	□	↑↓	↑	↑
Quinidine		⊘			□		□		□			→	↑	▦	↑↓	↑	↑
Propafenone		⊘						▦				↓	↓	□	↑	↑	
Flecainide			⊘		□							↓	→	□	↑	↑	
Bepridil	□			■	▦							↓		□			↑
Verapamil	□			■		▦						↓	↓	□	↑		
Diltiazem				▦								↓	↓	□	↑		
Bretylium				■			◐	◐				→	↓	□			↑
Amiodarone	□			□	■		▦	▦				→	↓	■	↑		↑
Nadolol								■				↓	↓	□	↑		
Propranolol	□							■				↓	↓	□	↑		
Atropine									■			→	↑	▦	↓		
Adenosine										○			↓	□			
Digoxin									○		■	↑	↓	■	↑		↓

relative potency of block: □ low ▦ moderate ■ high ⊘ = activated state blocker

○ = agonist ◐ = agonist/antagonist

Fig. 5.14 Spreadsheet approach to the classification of drugs (A₁, adenosine receptor; I_f, inward background depolarizing current of pacemaker caused by Na⁺ and Ca²⁺, termed "funny"; M₂, muscarinic receptor) (reproduced from *Eur Heart J* Vol 17, March 1996. Courtesy of W.B. Saunders Ltd.).

Disorders of the heart valves

Heart valve disease produces two types of disorders: stenosis and regurgitation. Stenosis is an obstruction to the normal flow of blood, whereas regurgitation (incompetence or reflux) is a failure of preventing the backflow of blood. Both conditions often coexist in the same valve (e.g., aortic stenosis and regurgitation after rheumatic fever).

Valvular disease can be caused by direct leaflet damage or by valve ring damage, or it may be secondary to damage of the papillary muscles or chordae. Major causes of acquired valve disease are as follows:

- Mitral stenosis—can be caused by rheumatic fever.

- Mitral regurgitation—can be caused by rheumatic fever, mitral valve prolapse, papillary muscle dysfunction, or valve ring dilatation.
- Aortic stenosis—can be caused by rheumatic fever or calcific degeneration.
- Aortic regurgitation—can be caused by rheumatic fever, aortic dilatation, or rheumatologic disorders.

Degenerative valve disease
Degenerative calcific aortic stenosis
Degenerative calcific aortic stenosis accounts for 90% of acquired aortic stenosis. This is an age-related degeneration, more common in the very old (aged over 70 years). Congenital bicuspid aortic valves (usually the valves are tricuspid) occur in 1% of the population. These valves become calcified much earlier in life (from about 50 years of age).

Rigid calcified deposits occur on the sinuses of Valsalva, resulting in thick, immobile valve cusps with narrowing of the orifice. Left ventricular hypertrophy usually results. Intervention is required if angina, syncope, or heart failure result.

Mitral annular calcification
Mitral annular calcification produces mitral regurgitation because the valve ring does not contract properly during systole. The condition also causes mitral stenosis because the bulky deposits prevent opening of the valves. Mitral annular calcification occurs more commonly in the elderly. Mitral stenosis increases the risk of thrombosis within the left atrium with subsequent systemic thromboembolism.

Calcific deposits may interfere with the conduction pathway, leading to arrhythmias, and they may also be a focus for infective endocarditis.

Myxomatous degeneration of the mitral valve (mitral valve prolapse)
Myxomatous degeneration causes billowing or prolapse of the mitral valve during systole, leading to regurgitation. The condition occurs in 15% of patients aged over 70 years. Cusps are thickened because of myxomatous (mucoid) deposition and fibrosis. Usually, this condition is asymptomatic except for a midsystolic click; an audible late systolic murmur indicates regurgitation. In severe disease, the chordae tendineae can rupture, causing sudden, severe regurgitation.

Rheumatic heart disease
Rheumatic heart disease is a consequence of rheumatic fever that may have occurred many years previously. The acute process can leave the valves scarred and deformed, causing chronic rheumatic heart disease. This occurs if the onset of acute rheumatic fever is in early childhood, is severe, and is chronic rheumatic fever.

Acute rheumatic fever
Acute rheumatic fever is an inflammatory disease caused by an autoimmune reaction initiated by infection with group A streptococci, usually in the throat. It mostly affects children aged 5–15 years. It is now extremely rare in the United States but continues to persist in patient populations from lower socioeconomic strata. It is common in the Middle East, Eastern Europe, the Far East, and South America.

It affects the heart, skin, joints, and central nervous system. Jones's criteria for diagnosis include:
- Carditis involving all three layers (pancarditis).
- Sydenham's chorea (St. Vitus dance: rapid, involuntary purposeless movements).
- Polyarthritis affecting the large joints.
- Erythema marginatum (macular rash with erythematous edge).
- Subcutaneous nodules.

Fever, arthralgia, and leukocytosis also commonly occur.

Carditis consists of granulomatous lesions with a central necrotic area (Aschoff body). Initially, there are macrophages, lymphocytes, and plasma cells, but these are replaced by fibrous scar tissue. On the valve, Aschoff bodies give rise to small vegetations (verrucae) of platelets and fibrin, which look like beads. Commonly, this affects the mitral valve (65%) or the mitral and aortic valves (25%). Recurrence is common if persistent carditis is present.

Chronic rheumatic fever
Chronic rheumatic fever is repeated attacks of rheumatic fever leading to chronic rheumatic heart disease, occurring in over half the patients with rheumatic carditis. This leads to commissural fusion, shortening/thickening of the chordae, and cusp fibrosis—the so-called "fish-mouth" or "button-hole" mitral valve deformity. Secondary changes in the heart occur as a result of:
- Mitral stenosis and regurgitation—leads to left atrial hypertrophy, pulmonary hypertension, atrial fibrillation, and thrombosis.

Acute compared with subacute manifestations of infective endocarditis		
Features	Acute	Subacute
Virulence of organism	High	Moderate or low
State of value before infection	Normal	Injured or abnormal
Type of infection	Necrotizing and invasive	Less destructive
Macroscopic vegetations	Larger and may cause emboli	Small to large
Presentation	Fever, rigors, malaise, splenomegaly, heart murmur	Low-grade fever, weight loss, flu-like syndrome, heart murmur
Course	Death occurs in 50% within days	Protracted course often less fatal

Fig. 5.15 Acute compared with subacute manifestations of infective endocarditis.

- Aortic stenosis—leads to left ventricular hypertrophy and arrhythmia.
- Aortic regurgitation—leads to left ventricular hypertrophy and dilatation.

Infective endocarditis

Infective endocarditis is an infection of the endocardium or vascular endothelium, usually involving the heart valves. In the past, it was classified as acute or subacute (Fig. 5.15); now it is classified according to the causative organism. The incidence is 2–5 per 100,000 in the United States, but it is more common in developing countries.

Infective endocarditis occurs more commonly on valves that have been previously damaged or are congenitally abnormal. Inflammation of the valve causes destruction and scarring.

Vegetations (consisting of fibrin, platelets, and the infecting organism) usually arise on the valves.

Causative agents include:
- *Streptococcus viridans*—subacute; common after dental procedures, tonsillectomy, or bronchoscopy.
- *Staphylococcus aureus*—acute; common in patients with indwelling catheters.
- *Enterococcus faecalis*—common in patients with pelvic infections or after having pelvic surgery.
- *Coxiella burnetii* (Q fever)—subacute.
- *Staphylococcus epidermidis, Aspergillus, Candida, Brucella, Histoplasma*—common in drug addicts and patients with prosthetic heart valves.

Sequelae of infective endocarditis include:
- Acute valve incompetence.
- Emboli to spleen, kidneys, and brain.
- Glomerulonephritis and renal failure.

Nonbacterial thrombotic (marantic) endocarditis

Marantic endocarditis causes small sterile fibrin and platelet thrombi on valves (mostly mitral) along the lines of closure. There is no inflammation or valvular damage. It usually occurs in cancer or a prolonged debilitating illness, and it is caused by a hypercoagulable state.

Endocarditis of systemic lupus erythematosus (Libman-Sacks disease)

Mitral and tricuspid valves are most commonly affected by Libman-Sacks disease. Fibrinoid necrosis, mucoid degeneration, and small vegetations on either side of the cusps may develop. Healing of vegetations may cause valve deformity.

Carcinoid heart disease

Carcinoid tumors (tumors of the enterochromaffin cells of the intestine) produce physiologically active substances (e.g., 5-hydroxytryptamine [serotonin], bradykinin, prostaglandins), which cause thickening of the tricuspid and pulmonary valves and parts of the right ventricle. The left side is usually unaffected.

101

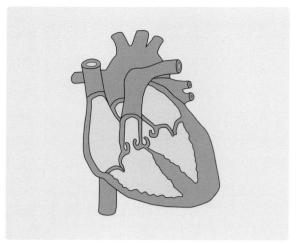

Fig. 5.16 A normal heart for comparison with the cardiomyopathic hearts shown in Figs. 5.17–5.19.

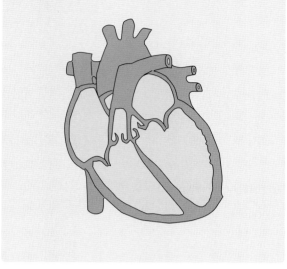

Fig. 5.17 Dilated cardiomyopathy. The ventricles are thin and dilated. Compare with Fig. 5.16.

Diseases of the myocardium

Myocardial disease can be categorized as either a cardiomyopathy or a specific heart muscle disease:
- A cardiomyopathy is any chronic disease affecting the muscle of the heart for which the cause is unknown (i.e., idiopathic, primary).
- Specific heart muscle disease is a disease for which the cause is known or associated with other disorders (e.g., alcoholic cardiomyopathy).

Myocardial dysfunction may also be a result of:
- Congenital heart disease.
- Hypertension.
- Ischemia.
- Valve disease.
- Pericardial disease.

Myocarditis is inflammation of the myocardium, and it is one of the main functional classes of specific heart muscle disease.

Cardiomyopathy

Cardiomyopathy is often functionally classified according to presentation into the following diseases:
- Dilated (congestive) cardiomyopathy (85%)—with dilated left ventricle and impaired systolic function.
- Hypertrophic (obstructive) cardiomyopathy (10%)—hypertrophy of ventricles, especially the interventricular septum; reduced diastolic filling.
- Restrictive cardiomyopathy (5%)—decreased ventricular compliance restricts ventricular filling.

Dilated cardiomyopathy

Dilated cardiomyopathy (Figs. 5.16 and 5.17) is associated with enlarged ventricular chambers and poor contraction. Its prevalence is approximately 0.2% in the general population.

Pathogenic factors include:
- Genetic defect.
- Alcohol toxicity.
- Postviral myocarditis—some myocarditis progresses to ventricular dilatation.
- Peripartum—may be caused by physiologic, pathologic, or metabolic changes in pregnancy.

Other associations include:
- Cardiovascular disease (e.g., ischemia, hypertension).
- Systemic disease (e.g., sarcoidosis, systemic lupus erythematosus).
- Neuromuscular disease (e.g., muscular dystrophy, Friedreich's ataxia).
- Glycogen storage disorder.
- Primary heart muscle disease (e.g., amyloidosis).
- Drug therapy: cytotoxic drugs (e.g., cyclophosphamide).

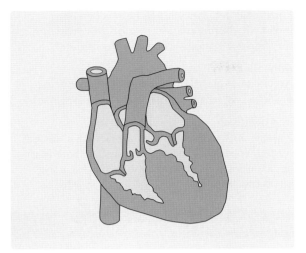

Fig. 5.18 Hypertrophic cardiomyopathy. There is an increase in ventricular mass. Compare with Fig. 5.16.

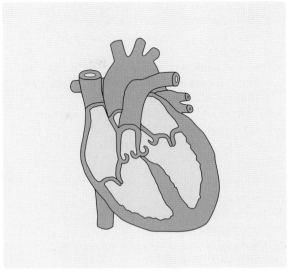

Fig. 5.19 Restrictive cardiomyopathy. The heart is of normal size, but the ventricles are stiff. Compare with Fig. 5.16.

The morphology of dilated cardiomyopathy is as follows:
- Cardiomegaly (up to 900 g), but dilated, thin walls in all chambers.
- Irregular myocyte hypertrophy and fibrosis.

Dilated cardiomyopathy can cause heart failure, arrhythmia, and emboli. Investigations include chest radiography, electrocardiography, and cardiac biopsy. Half of all patients diagnosed with dilated cardiomyopathies are under 65 years of age, and a quarter of those diagnosed present with symptoms consistent with New York Heart Association (NYHA) class III or IV heart disease.

Hypertrophic (obstructive) cardiomyopathy
Hypertrophic cardiomyopathy (HCM) (Fig. 5.18) is characterized by hypertrophy of the ventricles and septum; often it is asymmetrical. The disease causes distorted contraction and abnormal mitral valve movement. It is more common in young adults, and 50% of cases are inherited (autosomal dominant).
   The morphology of the hypertrophic cardiomyopathy is as follows:
- Asymmetric septal hypertrophy.
- Left ventricular cavity is banana-like.
- Myofiber hypertrophy and disarray.
- Patchy fibrosis.

Hypertrophic cardiomyopathy can also cause dyspnea, angina, syncope, and sudden death. Characteristic findings include a fourth heart sound,

a split early and late (bifid) carotid pulse, and systolic murmur. The course of the disease is very variable; many patients are unchanged for years.

Restrictive cardiomyopathy
Restrictive cardiomyopathy (Fig. 5.19) is a stiffening of the endomyocardium with restricted ventricular filling. It is the least common type of cardiomyopathy in the United States.
   Restrictive cardiomyopathy is often associated with:
- Amyloidosis—most common form in the United States.
- Endomyocardial fibrosis—most common in children and young adults in Africa.
- Löffler's endocarditis—found in temperate climates.

There is interstitial myocardial fibrosis (associated with eosinophilia in the latter two conditions). Dyspnea, fatigue, and emboli may be the presenting features. Symptoms are often similar to those seen in constrictive pericarditis.

Specific heart muscle disease
Myocarditis
Myocarditis is inflammation of the myocardium. Causes include:
- Infection—viruses (coxsackievirus, influenza, rubella, echovirus, polio); bacteria

(*Corynebacterium*—diphtheria, *Rickettsia*, *Chlamydia*); protozoa (*Trypanosoma cruzi*—Chagas' disease, *Toxoplasma gondii*); fungi (*Candida*).

- Immune-mediated reactions—after infections (viral or rheumatic fever); systemic lupus erythematosus; transplant rejection; chemicals, radiation, and drugs (chloroquine, methyldopa, lead poisoning).
- Idiopathic causes—sarcoidosis, giant cell myocarditis.

The morphology of myocarditis is as follows:
- Dilatation in all four chambers.
- Hemorrhagic mottling.
- Mural thrombi.
- Inflammatory infiltrate with focal myocyte necrosis and fibrosis.

Patients present with fever, dyspnea, angina, arrhythmia, and heart failure; the presentation is similar to myocardial infarction.

Other diseases

Other specific heart muscle diseases are generally associated with cardiotoxic agents, which cause myocyte swelling, fatty change, and lysis.

Fibrosis and scarring usually replace the focal lesions.

The various causes are explained below.

Alcohol

Alcohol causes a similar morphology to dilated cardiomyopathy. It may be associated with thiamine deficiency.

Adriamycin (doxorubicin) and other drugs

These cytotoxic drugs in toxic levels cause oxidation of the myocyte membranes, causing a similar morphology to dilated cardiomyopathy.

Catecholamines

Either exogenous (e.g., administered epinephrine) or endogenous (e.g., in pheochromocytoma) catecholamines can cause tachycardia and vasoconstriction, leading to patchy ischemic necrosis. This leads to a dilated cardiomyopathy. Cocaine may have a similar effect, because it inhibits norepinephrine reuptake.

Peripartum state

A dilated heart is found several months before and after delivery. The mechanism for this is uncertain, but it may include hypertension, volume overload, nutritional deficiency, immune reaction, or metabolic dysfunction. In 50% of these patients, function is restored several months later.

Amyloidosis

Amyloidosis may be systemic or isolated. It may produce arrhythmia or restrictive cardiomyopathy.

Iron overload

Patients with iron overload present with a dilated cardiomyopathy. This is often found in hereditary hemochromatosis and hemosiderosis (excessive blood transfusion).

Diseases of the pericardium

Fluid accumulation in the pericardial sac

Normally, the pericardial sac contains 50 mL of serous fluid. Its functions include:
- Lubrication.
- Prevention of sudden deformation or dislocation.
- A barrier to the spread of infection from the lungs.

Slow effusions allow greater volumes to accumulate before reaching the clinical threshold.

Pericardial effusion

A pericardial effusion:
- Is an accumulation of fluid in the pericardial cavity.
- Can be caused by any condition causing pericarditis.
- Can usually be morphologically classified as serous, serosanguineous, or chylous.

The effusion collects in the closed cavity and causes distension. When the pericardium cannot distend any more, pressure builds up, and cardiac tamponade results (impaired ventricular filling leading to loss of cardiac output).

Serous effusion

In a serous effusion, there is a smooth glistening serosa that secretes a watery fluid. It is usually a result of an inflammatory reaction and is common in most forms of acute pericarditis.

Serosanguineous effusion

These effusions are characterized by the presence of protein, including fibrinogen, in the exudate. They are usually characteristic of tubercular or neoplastic disease.

Chylous effusion

Chylous effusions are rare and are caused by lymphatic obstruction and leakage from the thoracic duct.

Hemopericardium

Hemopericardium is the accumulation of blood in the pericardial sac. It is caused by:

- Myocardial rupture after a myocardial infarction.
- Rupture of the aorta inside the pericardial sac.
- Hemorrhage from an abscess or tumor.
- Trauma.

If the accumulation of blood is greater than 200–300 mL, cardiac tamponade can result. Cardiac tamponade occurs when there is an abnormal external pressure on the heart. This impairs ventricular filling and affects cardiac output.

Clinical features of cardiac tamponade are heart failure, including a raised jugular venous pressure; Kussmaul's sign; exaggerated pulsus paradoxus; soft heart sounds; and an apex beat that may not be palpable. If a frictional rub is present, it may be quieter than before, because the fluid separates the parietal and visceral pericardium.

An echocardiogram is the best method for diagnosing a pericardial effusion.

Pericardial effusions may result in cardiac tamponade, which can quickly lead to reduced cardiac output and circulatory collapse. Thus, when signs of circulatory compromise arise, the pericardial space must be tapped (pericardiocentesis) to remove the excess fluid. These patients should be monitored carefully, because fluid often reaccumulates, especially if associated with tuberculosis or malignancy.

Cardiac tamponade is one of the causes of electromechanical dissociation. This occurs when the ventricular contraction is independent of the electrical activity of the heart (i.e., the electrical signal to contract is being sent to the ventricles, but no organized contraction occurs, and cardiac arrest results).

Electromechanical dissociation is an acute cardiorespiratory arrest, and it needs immediate treatment.

Other causes of electromechanical dissociation include:

- Tension pneumothorax.
- Hypovolemia.
- Massive pulmonary embolism.

Common causes of pericarditis	
Cause	**Pathology**
Viral (coxsackievirus)	Fibrinous
Myocardial infarction	Fibrinous and may lead to fibrous adhesions
Uremia	Fibrinous
Carcinoma (metastatic spread, often from the lung)	Serous or hemorrhagic
Connective tissue disease (rheumatic fever)	Fibrinous
Bacterial	Purulent
Tuberculosis	Caseous
After cardiac surgery	Fibrinous
Diester syndrome (after a myocardial infarction)	Autoimmune

Fig. 5.20 Common causes of pericarditis.

- Drug overdose.
- Hypothermia.

Pericarditis

Pericarditis is an inflammation of the pericardium leading to sharp substernal chest pain that radiates to the back and that is aggravated by movement and respiration. Common causes are listed in Fig. 5.20.

Acute pericarditis

Commonly, acute pericarditis is caused by an acute viral (coxsackievirus) infection or a myocardial infarction. Morphologically acute pericarditis can be separated into the following categories:

- Serous—slowly accumulating serous exudate with inflammatory cells.
- Fibrinous/serofibrinous—most common, may resolve completely or leave adhesions.
- Suppurative (purulent)—bacterial/fungal infection with pus; may produce constrictive pericarditis.
- Hemorrhagic—blood exudate with fibrin or pus; may calcify.
- Caseous—leads to constrictive pericarditis; caused by tuberculosis.

Chronic pericarditis

Healing of pericarditis can result in complete resolution, thick plaques, or adhesions.

Adhesive pericarditis

In adhesive pericarditis, the parietal pericardium becomes attached to the mediastinum, and the pericardial sac no longer exists. The heart dilates and hypertrophies.

Constrictive pericarditis

In constrictive pericarditis, there is a thick, fibrous, often calcified pericardial sac that encases the heart, limiting cardiac filling and reducing cardiac output. Symptoms of heart failure result.

Rheumatic disease of the pericardium

Pericarditis occurs in 30% of people with severe chronic rheumatoid arthritis. Granulomas may lead to fibrous adhesions, causing constrictive pericarditis.

Inflammatory vascular disease

Concepts and classification

The vasculitides are a group of conditions characterized by vasculitis (inflammation and damage of the vessel walls) (Fig. 5.21). They may be classified by pathogenesis (infective, immune-mediated, or idiopathic) or by the size of the vessel affected (large, medium, or small).

Most systemic vasculitides probably involve an immunologic process. Many different processes have been described. There may be deposition of circulating antigen-antibody complexes in conditions such as systemic lupus erythematosus. Antibodies may react with fixed tissue antigens as in Kawasaki syndrome. Temporal arteritis involves delayed-type hypersensitivity reactions with granuloma formation.

The presence of antineutrophilic cytoplasmic autoantibodies (ANCA), which react with antigens in the cytoplasm of neutrophils, can be seen in many vasculitides. The antigen may be perinuclear (p-ANCA) or cytoplasmic (c-ANCA).

Infectious vasculitides

The causes of infectious vasculitides may be:
- Bacterial (e.g., *Neisseria*).
- Viral (e.g., herpes).
- Other infectious causes such as *Rickettsia* (Rocky Mountain spotted fever), spirochetes (syphilis), or fungi (*Aspergillus*).

Immunologic vasculitides

The immunologic vasculitides can be classified as:
- Immune-complex—Henoch–Schönlein purpura, systemic lupus erythematosus.
- Direct antibody—Goodpasture's syndrome (anti–basement membrane antibodies), Kawasaki disease.
- ANCA-associated—Wegener's granulomatosis, microscopic polyarteritis.
- Cell-mediated—organ rejection.

Idiopathic vasculitides
Giant-cell (temporal) arteritis

Giant-cell arteritis is the most common of the vasculitides, occurring in the elderly and being rare in those younger than 55 years of age. There is focal granulomatous inflammation of medium and small arteries, especially the cranial vessels. It usually presents with headache, facial pain, and polymyalgia rheumatica (flu-like aches and fever). The erythrocyte sedimentation ratio (ESR) and/or C reactive protein (CRP) are usually raised. Visual disturbances develop in about half of affected individuals and may lead to blindness without prompt intervention.

Diagnosis is by temporal artery biopsy; microscopically, the following signs are seen:
- Granulations with giant cells.
- General leukocytic infiltrate.
- Fibrosis of the intima and stenosis.

Vessels affected by vasculitides		
Vessel size	**Arteries**	**Disease**
Large/ medium	Aorta Carotid Temporal	Giant cell arteritis, Takayasu's arteritis
Medium/ small	Coronary Mesenteric	Polyarteritis nodosa, Kawasaki disease
Small/ arteriole	Glomeruli and arterioles	Wegener's granulomatosis, microscopic polyarteritis nodosa
Arteriole/ capillary	–	Henoch-Schönlein purpura, Cutaneous leukocytoclastic
Veins	–	Buerger's disease

Fig. 5.21 Vessels affected by vasculitides.

There is often associated thrombosis. Biopsy may be negative in one third of cases. Treatment is with corticosteroids.

Takayasu's disease (aortic arch syndrome)

Takayasu's disease typically affects females in the 20- to 40-year-old age group. It is most common in Asia. It is a granulomatous vasculitis of medium-to-large arteries, especially the aorta and the great vessels. Patients present with visual disturbances, neurologic deficits, and diminished upper pulses ("pulseless disease"). If the renal arteries are involved, hypertension may result. There is thickening of the aortic wall with mononuclear cell infiltrates. Fibrosis and granulomas may result.

Polyarteritis nodosa

Polyarteritis nodosa is twice as common in males as in females, usually occurring in middle age. It is associated with the hepatitis B surface (s) antigen. p-ANCA may have a role.

Fibrinoid necrosis of medium-to-small arteries occurs, especially of the main viscera (e.g., coronary, renal, and hepatic arteries). The pulmonary arteries are not usually affected. Presenting features can be general (e.g., fever) or relate to the system involved:
- Renal—hypertension, renal failure.
- Cardiac—myocardial infarction, heart failure.
- Central nervous system—hemiplegia, psychoses.
- Gastrointestinal—abdominal pain, melena.

Segmental lesions occur, with fibrinoid necrosis of the wall and a neutrophil infiltrate. Healing results in thickening and aneurysmal dilatation. A type of polyarteritis nodosa known as Churg–Strauss syndrome affects the lungs. Diagnosis is by biopsy; treatment is with antiviral therapy for hepatitis B-associated polyarteritis or immunosuppression.

Kawasaki syndrome (mucocutaneous lymph node syndrome)

Kawasaki syndrome is an acute febrile illness of young children. Patients present with lymphadenopathy, rash, erythema, peeling skin, and (in 20% of those affected) coronary arteritis with aneurysms, which may lead to myocardial infarction or sudden cardiac death.

Similar lesions occur to those seen in polyarteritis nodosa. Aspirin and γ-globulin therapy are thought to prevent cardiac complications.

Microscopic polyarteritis (leukocytoclastic angiitis)

Microscopic polyarteritis is a fibrinoid necrosis of the smallest vessels, and it is thought to be a form of hypersensitivity reaction. Typically, there is an acute onset with a precipitating agent (e.g., bacteria) and involvement of the skin or viscera. There may be little neutrophilic infiltrate.

Wegener's granulomatosis

This represents the majority of cases in patients aged over 50 years. The condition consists of a triad of symptoms:
- Necrotizing vasculitis of the lung and upper respiratory tract.
- Granulomas of the respiratory tract.
- Glomerulonephritis of the kidneys.

c-ANCA type autoantibodies are usually present. Lesions are similar to those of polyarteritis nodosa, but granulomas also occur. Treatment is by immunosuppression (using prednisolone and cyclophosphamide).

Thromboangiitis obliterans (Buerger's disease)

Thromboangiitis obliterans is typically found in male smokers aged under 35 years. It is twice as common in Jews than in non-Jews. It involves inflammation of the vessels of the lower limbs. Nodular phlebitis (inflammation of veins) and ischemia of the extremities result. There is neutrophilic infiltration with thrombi and giant-cell formation.

Frequently, the condition is painful and leads to gangrene if smoking is not stopped.

Vasculitis in systemic disease

Many diseases have vasculitis as a component.

Systemic lupus erythematosus

Systemic lupus erythematosus (SLE) affects capillaries, arterioles, and venules. An inflammatory vasculitis is predominant; neutrophils are more common than lymphocytes. Vasculitic lesions on the skin, muscle, and brain are common. Raynaud's phenomenon may also be present. A similar pathology exists in other connective tissue disorders (e.g., scleroderma, cryoglobulinemia).

Henoch–Schönlein purpura

This is a hypersensitivity reaction that is often preceded by infection. Purpuric rashes caused by inflammation of capillaries and venules are present on the legs and buttocks. Abdominal pain, arthritis, hematuria, and nephritis may also occur.

Rheumatoid vasculitis

Vasculitis is one of the extra-articular features of rheumatoid arthritis.

Infectious vasculitis

Systemic infections can result in a vasculitis. These often produce a purpuric rash due to a hypersensitivity reaction.

Raynaud's disease

Raynaud's disease is not strictly a vasculitis, but it is worth considering here, because it has some features in common with other vasculitides.

Raynaud's disease affects 5% of the population, and it is mainly found in young healthy women. There is pallor and cyanosis caused by vasospasm of the small arteries/arterioles in the hands and feet. The exact etiology is unknown, but it is thought to be due to increased vasomotor responses to cold or emotion.

Raynaud's phenomenon refers to the decrease in blood flow that occurs secondary to the narrowing of the arteries that supply the extremities. It implies a known etiology; this can be atherosclerosis, systemic lupus erythematosus, scleroderma, or Buerger's disease.

Congenital abnormalities of the heart

Congenital heart defects have an incidence of 6–8 per 1000 liveborn infants. They may present in the first year of life or remain asymptomatic for life.

Left-to-right shunts

Left-to-right shunts very rarely cause cyanosis at birth; thus, they are collectively termed "acyanotic" lesions.

Atrial septal defect

An atrial septal defect (ASD) is caused by a failure of proper closure of the foramen ovale or by a defect in the septum secundum (Fig. 5.22). Blood moves from the left atrium into the right atrium because of the pressure difference. Atrial septal defects make up 10% of all congenital heart defects.

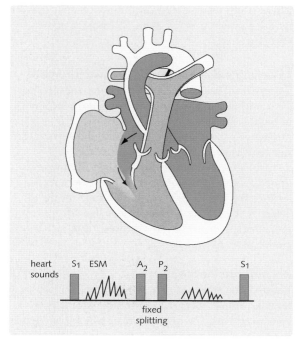

Fig. 5.22 Atrial septal defect (S_1, first heart sound from closure of mitral and tricuspid valves; A_2, heart sound from closure of aortic valve; ESM, ejection systolic murmur; P_2, heart sound from closure of pulmonary valve) (from *Illustrated Textbook of Paediatrics*, 2nd ed. by Lissauer T, Clayden G, London, Mosby, 2001).

Frequently, the child is asymptomatic, but clinical features can include:
- Recurrent chest infections, heart failure, and arrhythmias.
- Fixed, widely split second heart sound.
- Ejection systolic murmur, best heard in the third intercostal space, produced by increased flow across the pulmonary valve (left-to-right shunt).

Electrocardiography, chest radiography, and echocardiography will confirm the diagnosis. In children with symptoms, treatment is by a catheter-delivered device or surgery.

Ventricular septal defect

A ventricular septal defect (VSD) is a failure of fusion of the interventricular septum or endocardial cushions (Fig. 5.23). Blood shunts through a hole in the interventricular septum.

Ventricular septal defects make up 30% of all congenital heart lesions. The patient may be asymptomatic, but clinical features can include:

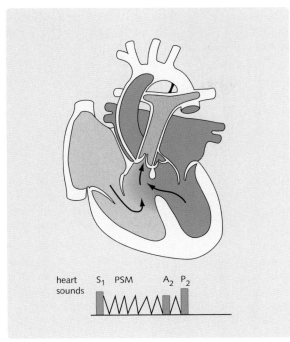

Fig. 5.23 Ventricular septal defect (S_1, first heart sound from closure of mitral and tricuspid valves; A_2, heart sound from closure of aortic valve; PSM, pansystolic murmur; P_2, heart sound from closure of pulmonary valve) (from *Illustrated Textbook of Paediatrics*, 2nd ed. by Lissauer T, Clayden G, London, Mosby, 2001).

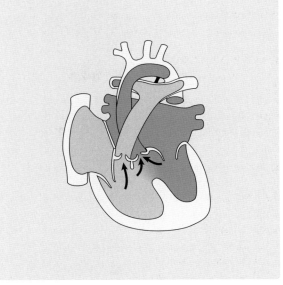

Fig. 5.24 Eisenmenger's syndrome. The shunt has reversed (and now goes from right to left). Less blood now goes into the pulmonary trunk, and the patient becomes cyanotic (from *Illustrated Textbook of Paediatrics*, 2nd ed. by Lissauer T, Clayden G, London, Mosby, 2001).

- Heart failure, failure to thrive, recurrent chest infections.
- Palpable parasternal thrill.
- Loud pansystolic murmur at lower left sternal edge.

Electrocardiography, echocardiography, and chest radiography will confirm the diagnosis.

Most ventricular septal defects will close spontaneously within the first 2 years of life. However, 10% will require surgical repair.

If there is a large left-to-right shunt, there will be a great deal of blood entering the right ventricle and pulmonary circulation, causing pulmonary hypertension. Eventually, the pulmonary hypertension will cause irreversible damage to the pulmonary vasculature. This will cause right ventricular hypertrophy, which may eventually lead to reversal of the shunt from right to left. This is called Eisenmenger's syndrome and often leads to cyanosis (Fig. 5.24).

Other large left-to-right shunts (e.g., atrial septal defects or patent ductus arteriosus) can also lead to Eisenmenger's syndrome.

Patent ductus arteriosus

Patent ductus arteriosus is caused by an open ductus arteriosus, which allows the communication of blood between the systemic and pulmonary circulations (Fig. 5.25). It accounts for 10% of all congenital heart defects.

There is a continuous murmur beneath the left clavicle and a collapsing pulse.

Echocardiography is the most useful investigation.

In preterm infants, the duct usually will ultimately close, but closure with indomethacin (inhibits prostaglandin production) or with a catheter-delivered device may be required.

Infective endocarditis may result if the duct never closes.

Atrioventricular septal defect

An atrioventricular septal defect (AVSD) results from failure of the superior and inferior endocardial cushions to fuse (Fig. 5.26). Surgical repair is complex and hazardous. Obstruction of the left

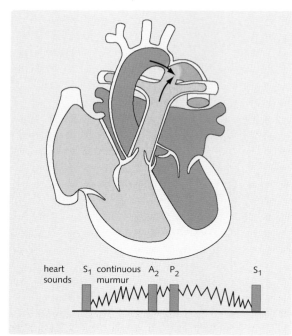

Fig. 5.25 Patent ductus arteriosus. This is often found with coarctation of the aorta (shown). It allows mixing of systemic and pulmonary blood. Movement of blood within the ductus can occur in both directions, depending upon the relative pressures in the aorta and the pulmonary trunk (S_1, first heart sound from closure of mitral and tricuspid valves; A_2, heart sound from closure of aortic valve; P_2, heart sound from closure of pulmonary valve) (from *Illustrated Textbook of Paediatrics* by Lissauer T, Clayden G, London, Mosby, 1997).

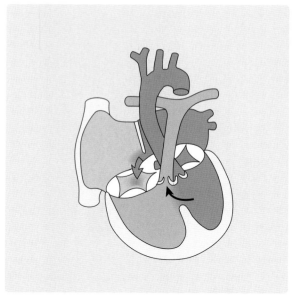

Fig. 5.26 Atrioventricular septal defect (AVSD). There is very little separation between the atria and ventricles (from *Illustrated Textbook of Paediatrics* by Lissauer T, Clayden G, London, Mosby, 1997).

ventricular outflow tract is one long-term consequence.

Right-to-left shunts

Right-to-left shunts commonly cause cyanosis. Thus, they are collectively termed "cyanotic" lesions.

Tetralogy of Fallot

Tetralogy of Fallot (Fig. 5.27) is a combination of:
- Large ventricular septal defect.
- Pulmonary stenosis.
- Right ventricular hypertrophy.
- Aorta overriding the interventricular septum.

The tetralogy occurs in 6% of children with heart defects. Severe cyanosis with hypercyanotic episodes may result. A loud ejection systolic murmur is heard in the third left intercostal space, and finger clubbing may develop. Corrective surgery is required, which can be started at 4–6 months of age.

Transposition of the great arteries

Transposition of the great arteries occurs when the truncoconal septum develops, but it does not spiral (Fig. 5.28). The left ventricle pumps blood into the pulmonary trunk, and the right ventricle pumps blood into the aorta. There is usually also an atrial septal defect, ventricular septal defect, or patent ductus arteriosus to allow blood to mix; otherwise, this would be incompatible with life.

Transposition of the great arteries occurs in 4% of cardiac defects. Severe cyanosis may result. There may be finger clubbing and various murmurs. Ultimately, surgical treatment is required.

Persistent truncus arteriosus

The truncoconal septum fails to form, leading to a common outflow tract for both ventricles. There is also a ventricular septal defect in this very rare condition.

Tricuspid atresia

In tricuspid atresia, there is an absence of the tricuspid valve, causing poor pulmonary circulation. The neonate has a duct-dependent circulation (i.e., other communications are needed between the arterial and venous systems to prevent serious

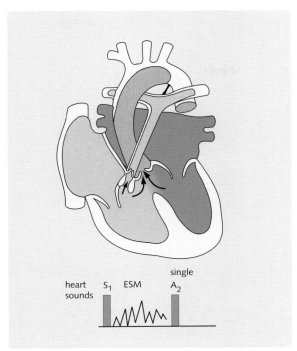

heart sounds S_1 ESM   single A_2

Fig. 5.27 Tetralogy of Fallot. The right-to-left shunt that results causes cyanosis (S_1, first heart sound from closure of mitral and tricuspid valves; A_2, heart sound from closure of aortic valve; ESM, ejection systolic murmur) (from *Illustrated Textbook of Paediatrics*, 2nd ed. by Lissauer T, Clayden G, London, Mosby, 2001).

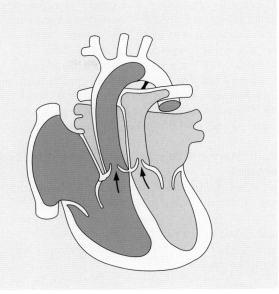

Fig. 5.28 Transposition of the great arteries. This is incompatible with life without a ventricular (VSD) or atrial septal defect (ASD) or a patent ductus arteriosus (from *Illustrated Textbook of Paediatrics*, 2nd ed. by Lissauer T, Clayden G, London, Mosby, 2001).

cyanosis). Surgery is required to replace the tricuspid valve.

Obstructive congenital defects
Coarctation of the aorta

Coarctation of the aorta is a narrowing of the aorta in the area of the ductus arteriosus (Fig. 5.29). The narrowing may occur either proximal to the ductus (preductal coarctation) or distal to the ductus (distal coarctation). The location makes a significant difference in the clinical presentation of the patient. Preductal coarctation develops in utero and is associated with a poorly formed and hypoplastic aorta. These patients often present shortly after birth with congestive heart failure and a characteristic pattern of "differential cyanosis" in which the upper body is normally perfused by vessels arising from the ascending aorta, but the lower body is cyanotic because vessels beyond the point of coarctation must be supplied by "venous" blood flowing from the right side of the heart via a patent ductus arteriosus.

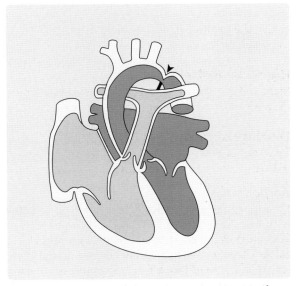

Fig. 5.29 Coarctation of the aorta, causing stenosis (from *Illustrated Textbook of Paediatrics*, 2nd ed. by Lissauer T, Clayden G, London, Mosby, 2001).

Postductal coarctation is associated with elevated left ventricular pressures and may lead to heart failure if the coarctation is severe. These patients usually do not present with cyanosis. Taken together, coarctation of the aorta represents about 7% of congenital heart defects. Common clinical findings include weak or absent femoral pulses, a systolic ejection murmur, and upper extremity hypertension. Surgical intervention is frequently required.

Pulmonary stenosis with intact interventricular septum

Of those children with heart defects, 7% present with a stenosis of the pulmonary valve (Fig. 5.30); most are asymptomatic. An ejection systolic murmur and ejection click may be heard. Treatment is indicated when right ventricular hypertrophy occurs or the stenosis worsens.

Link the problems that can occur in embryologic development with the pressure changes that occur in the cardiac cycle to work out what sort of shunting mechanism occurs with each defect. Also, any shunt that occurs is going to cause turbulent flow, so the timing of the shunt in the cardiac cycle will tell you what type of murmur occurs. For example, a ventricular septal defect is a defect in the development of the interventricular septum. The left ventricular pressure is greater than the right because of its larger muscle mass; therefore, blood is going to flow from left to right. As this shunt occurs throughout systole, a pansystolic murmur occurs.

Aortic stenosis

Stenosis of the aortic valve occurs in 6% of neonates with heart defects (Fig. 5.31). Usually, there is associated mitral stenosis and coarctation of the aorta. There may be heart failure, syncope, and chest pain. Clinical features also include slow-rising pulses, an ejection click, and ejection systolic murmur. Eventually, surgical repair and valve replacement are necessary.

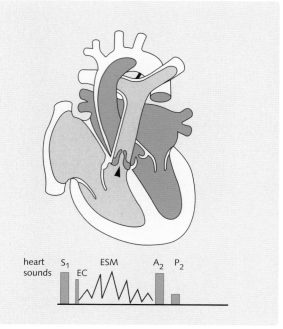

Fig. 5.30 Pulmonary stenosis (S_1, first heart sound from closure of mitral and tricuspid valves; A_2, heart sound from closure of aortic valve; EC, ejection click; ESM, ejection systolic murmur; P_2, heart sound from closure of pulmonary valve) (from *Illustrated Textbook of Paediatrics*, 2nd ed. by Lissauer T, Clayden G, London, Mosby, 2001).

Congenital abnormalities of the vessels

Vascular anatomy is complex, and it undergoes considerable remodeling during embryologic development. There are many areas in which departures from the usual development can occur. These do not necessarily produce deficiencies in the flow of blood; rather, most represent an alternative supply and drainage of the same tissue. For example, errors in the remodeling of the great vessels may give rise to double inferior and superior venae cavae. This is caused by a failure of regression of a primitive element.

A vascular ring may form around the esophagus and trachea, causing difficulty in swallowing and breathing. This is caused by a persistent right dorsal aorta, or it may result from other problems in aortic arch development.

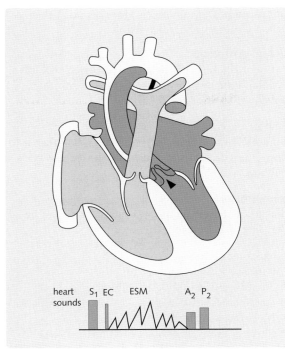

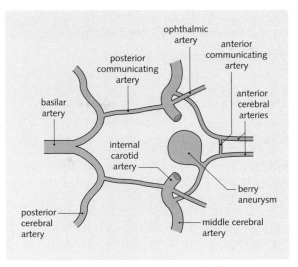

Fig. 5.32 Berry aneurysm in the circle of Willis.

Fig. 5.31 Aortic stenosis (S_1, first heart sound from closure of mitral and tricuspid valves; A_2, heart sound from closure of aortic valve; EC, ejection click; ESM, ejection systolic murmur; P_2, heart sound from closure of pulmonary valve) (from *Illustrated Textbook of Paediatrics*, 2nd ed. by Lissauer T, Clayden G, London, Mosby, 2001).

Lymphedema may result from hypoplasia of the lymphatic system.

Abnormalities in the coronary circulation may sometimes be normal (e.g., when branches of the left coronary artery arise directly from the aorta), or they may lead to ischemia and infarction of the myocardium.

Two important anomalies of the circulation are:
- Arteriovenous fistulas.
- Berry aneurysms.

Arteriovenous fistula

An arteriovenous fistula is an abnormal communication between an artery and a vein. This may be congenital in origin or secondary to trauma, inflammation, or a healed ruptured aneurysm. Fistulas may cause shunting of blood, bypassing circulations and increasing venous return, thereby increasing cardiac output. This may predispose to heart failure.

Fistulas may be seen in Paget's disease of the bone, where the increased blood flow through the affected bones may eventually lead to heart failure.

Arteriovenous fistulas are used in hemodialysis for renal patients. Artificial arteriovenous fistulas can be surgically placed between the radial artery and cephalic vein. This causes the vein to distend and thicken, enabling large bore needles to be inserted. These take blood to and from the dialysis machine.

Berry aneurysm

Berry aneurysms are found in about 2% of postmortem examinations, and they are the most common intracranial aneurysm. They are small saccular aneurysms in the cerebral vessels. They can measure about 0.2–3.0 cm in diameter but are usually around 1.0 cm. They frequently occur at branch points in the circle of Willis (Fig. 5.32). These aneurysms are commonly seen in patients with coarctation of the aorta and polycystic renal disease.

Berry aneurysms are asymptomatic until they rupture (usually when the patient is aged between 40 and 60 years). Rupture is more common in males. Predisposing factors to rupture include smoking, hypertension, and atheroma. The original outpouching is caused by local focal wall weakness. This then gets larger as a result of luminal hemodynamics. Eventually, rupture may occur. Rupture of berry aneurysms results in a subarachnoid hemorrhage. This presents with a sudden onset of severe headache, and it may be fatal.

Neoplastic heart disease

Primary cardiac tumors

Primary cardiac tumors include myxoma, lipoma, papillary fibroelastoma, rhabdomyoma, and sarcoma. They are extremely rare.

Myxoma

Myxomas account for 25% of primary cardiac tumors. Presentation can be at any age, but mostly it occurs in adults; 75% of myxomas occur in the left atrium. They can be polyploid or pedunculated masses, arising from undifferentiated connective tissue in the subendocardial layer. If pedunculated, the tumor mass may have limited movement within the heart chamber, sufficient to periodically occlude cardiac outflow (ball-valve obstruction). Of patients with myxoma, 50% show signs and symptoms of mitral valve disease. Myxomatous masses can fragment and produce emboli.

Lipoma

Lipomas usually occur in the interatrial septum. They are well circumscribed, poorly encapsulated adipose tissue.

Papillary fibroelastoma

Papillary fibroelastomas are filamentous projections found in right-sided valves in children and left-sided valves in adults. They are composed of connective tissue with smooth muscle and fibroblasts.

Rhabdomyoma

Many rhabdomyomas occur in neonates, causing stillbirth or death in the first few days of life. They are often multiple, and they arise from cardiac muscle. They have strands in the cytoplasm radiating out of the nucleus, and so they are called spider cells.

Sarcoma

Malignant tumors include rhabdomyosarcomas and angiosarcomas.

Cardiovascular effects of neoplastic disease
Direct effects
Metastases

Metastases that develop in the myocardium are usually from bronchial carcinomas or malignant melanomas. They are much more common than primary tumors of cardiac tissue.

Vessel obstruction

A tumor can obstruct neighboring vessels by local invasion into vessel walls, compression by growth outside the vessel, and by producing emboli.

Emboli

Tumors can fragment and send off emboli that will impact in a vessel (e.g., a tumor in the leg may cause a pulmonary embolus).

Hemorrhage

Malignant tumors on mucosa can ulcerate and bleed. Bleeding can also occur into a tumor.

Circulating factors

Circulating factors can lead to:
- Nonbacterial thrombotic endocarditis.
- Carcinoid heart disease.
- Myeloma-associated amyloidosis.
- Pheochromocytoma-associated heart disease.

Iatrogenic effects of therapy

There are many unwanted effects of therapy of neoplastic disease. Radiotherapy causes lethargy, appetite loss, and rashes, for example. Chemotherapy causes nausea, vomiting, alopecia, and marrow suppression. Each modality and substance has its own specific side effects. Surgical therapy can be risky and complicated, especially because some tissues are highly vascularized. However, there are few general iatrogenic effects that affect the cardiovascular system.

Neoplastic vascular disease

Benign tumors and related conditions
Hemangioma

Hemangiomas are common, especially in children; they make up approximately 7% of all benign tumors. Hemangiomas are usually subdivided into capillary hemangiomas, juvenile capillary hemangiomas, cavernous hemangiomas, and granuloma pyogenicum.

Capillary hemangioma

Capillary hemangiomas occur mostly in skin and mucous membranes. These are well-defined, encapsulated aggregates of capillaries. They may be thrombosed.

Juvenile capillary ("strawberry") hemangioma

Juvenile capillary hemangiomas are present at birth on the face and scalp of infants. They grow rapidly for the first few months, then regress and disappear by the age of 5 years.

Cavernous hemangioma

Cavernous hemangiomas are large, cavernous, vascular channels that are not encapsulated. They involve skin, mucous membranes, the central nervous system, and the liver.

Granuloma pyogenicum

Granuloma pyogenicum is an ulcerated version of capillary hemangioma, often caused by trauma. Typically, it is composed of capillaries with edema, inflammatory cells, and granulation tissue. Granuloma gravidum occurs in the gums of up to 5% of pregnant women.

Glomangioma

Glomangiomas are painful tumors of the glomus body (a receptor in the smooth muscle of arteries that is sensitive to temperature [i.e., at arteriovenous anastomoses in the skin]). Glomangiomas are usually found in fingers or nail beds. They are branching vascular channels with aggregates of glomus bodies.

Telangiectasias

Telangiectasias are aggregations of prominent small vessels in the skin or mucous membranes. They are probably not a true neoplasm, but are either congenital or an exaggeration of existing vessels.

Nevus flammeus (ordinary birthmark)

Nevus flammeus is a macular lesion with vessel dilatation. Most regress, except the "port-wine stain" nevi, which persist and are a sign of the Sturge–Weber syndrome.

Spider nevi (nevus araneus)

Spider nevi are minute, often pulsatile arterioles occurring around a central core, usually above the waist. They are associated with hyperestrogen states (e.g., cirrhosis and pregnancy).

Rendu-Osler-Weber disease (hereditary hemorrhagic telangiectasia)

Rendu-Osler-Weber disease is a rare autosomal dominant condition, characterized by multiple small aneurysms on the skin and mucous membranes. Patients present with bleeding from the nose, mouth, or rectum, or in urine.

Bacillary angiomatosis

Bacillary angiomatosis is a potentially fatal disease if left untreated. It is caused by rickettsia-like bacteria. There is proliferation of blood vessels in the skin, lymph nodes, and organs of immunocompromised patients. Treatment with erythromycin is curative.

Intermediate-grade tumors

Hemangioendothelioma

Hemangioendotheliomas are neoplasms that show both benign and malignant characteristics (i.e., some are benign, others are malignant). They consist of vascular channels with masses of spindle-shaped plump cells of endothelial origin.

Malignant tumors

Angiosarcoma (hemangiosarcoma)

Angiosarcomas are rare but very aggressive tumors that metastasize widely. They are found in skin, breasts, the liver, and the spleen, especially in the elderly. There are small, discrete, red nodules that change into large, white masses, in which cells of all differentiations are found.

Hemangiopericytoma

Hemangiopericytoma is a malignant tumor of pericytes occurring in the lower extremities or in the retroperitoneum. About half of all these tumors metastasize.

Kaposi's sarcoma

Kaposi's sarcoma is a malignant tumor of unknown origin, but it is probably from lymphatic endothelium. Purple papules/plaques are found in the skin, mucosa, or viscera. Microscopically, it is composed of sheets of spindle-shaped plump cells with intermingled red blood cells and vascular channels.

There are four types of this disease. Their descriptions follow.

Classic Kaposi's sarcoma

Classic Kaposi's sarcoma affects mainly elderly Eastern European men, especially Ashkenazi Jews. Multiple red plaques occur on the lower extremities. The disease is rarely fatal.

African Kaposi's sarcoma

African Kaposi's sarcoma affects mainly younger men in equatorial Africa. Clinically, it is similar to classic Kaposi's sarcoma.

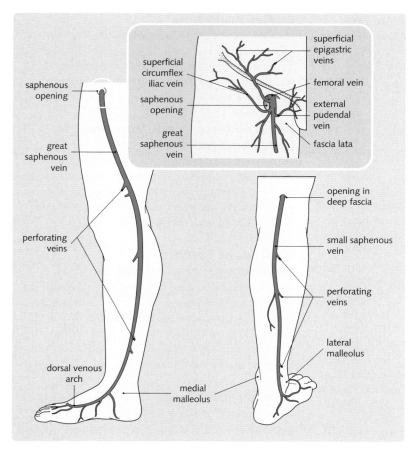

Fig. 5.33 Perforating veins of the lower limbs.

Transplant-associated Kaposi's sarcoma

Transplant-associated Kaposi's sarcoma occurs in immunosuppressed patients. It involves the skin and viscera. Lesions regress when immunosuppression is stopped.

HIV-associated Kaposi's sarcoma

HIV-associated Kaposi's sarcoma may occur in the skin, mucous membranes, lymph nodes, viscera, or gastrointestinal tract. This is an AIDS-defining illness, and it often responds to cytotoxic drugs or α-interferon.

Diseases of the veins and lymphatics

Varicose veins

Varicose veins are tortuous, distended superficial veins, usually of the lower limbs, caused by a persistent increased intraluminal pressure. They

occur in 10–20% of the normal population, with women being more affected than men. Risk factors include:

- Pregnancy.
- Obesity.
- Prolonged standing.
- Previous deep vein thrombosis.
- Familial tendency.
- Tumors compressing the deep veins.

Etiology

There are superficial and deep veins in the lower limb, which are interconnected by perforating veins (Fig. 5.33). Blood is returned mainly through the deep veins to the thoracic compartment by the skeletal pumping effect of the calf muscles. If there is a blockage of the deep veins (e.g., by thrombosis) or if there are faulty valves in the perforating veins, then blood will move from the deep veins into the superficial veins. This will lead to distension and further valvular incompetence, resulting in stasis of blood. Edema and changes in the skin take place (e.g., ulceration, which fails to heal because there is an impaired circulation).

Histologically, the venous walls will become thin where there is dilatation. Thrombosis may be seen in the superficial vein walls, but this rarely causes emboli.

Sequelae

Sequelae of varicose veins include:
- Varicose ulcers.
- Dermatitis.
- Thromboemboli.

Other parts of the body where varicosities may occur

- Hemorrhoids are distended submucosal veins in the anal canal that may protrude through the anus. Bleeding and pain may result from trauma, protrusion, or spasm of the anal sphincter.
- Varicocele is a distension of the veins of the pampiniform plexus in the spermatic cord.
- Esophageal varices are distended veins at the esophageal-gastric junction. They are caused by portal hypertension, usually as a result of hepatic cirrhosis.

Phlebothrombosis and thrombophlebitis

Thrombosis within a vein is termed "phlebothrombosis"—the term "deep vein thrombosis" is more specific. Phlebothrombosis usually causes inflammation in the wall of the vein, which is then termed "thrombophlebitis." Risk factors for thrombosis include:
- Pregnancy.
- Prolonged immobilization.
- Surgery (i.e., leading to immobilization).
- Tumor.
- Local infection.
- Congestive heart failure.
- Dehydration.

Thrombosis mainly affects the following:
- Deep leg veins (90% of thromboses; 60% of hospitalized patients on autopsy). Commonly, they throw off emboli that lodge in the pulmonary circulation.

- Periprostatic plexus in men.
- Ovarian and pelvic veins in women.

Clinical features of thrombosis vary:
- It may be asymptomatic.
- It may present with pulmonary emboli.
- It may cause calf pain, with swelling, redness, and distended superficial veins. The affected calf is warmer, and there may be ankle edema.
- If severe, occlusion may lead to cyanosis of the limb, severe edema, and gangrene.

Investigation is with Doppler ultrasonography or venography. Treatment is by anticoagulation therapy with heparin. The patient is mobilized and advised to wear support stockings.

In late pregnancy, phlegmasia alba dolens (painful white "milk leg") may occur because of thrombosis of the iliofemoral veins.

Thrombophlebitis migrans (Trousseau's syndrome) refers to multiple thrombi occurring in one place and then vanishing only to occur somewhere else. It is caused by hypercoagulability states associated with cancer.

 Deep vein thrombosis is often asymptomatic, but it may lead to fatal complications. Any immobile patient should be considered at risk. Long-haul flights are a risk factor, even for young adults. Fluid intake, aspirin, and regular leg exercise will minimize risk.

Lymphangitis and lymphedema

Lymphangitis is inflammation of the lymphatic vessels. It is frequently found in lymphatic vessels that drain a source of infection. It often presents as a cluster of red painful streaks in the skin close to an infected site. Lymphangitis very often occurs as a result of bacterial infections (especially streptococcal). If untreated with antibiotics, it may progress to involve the lymph nodes (lymphadenitis), and it may eventually lead to septicemia.

Histologically, the wall of the affected lymph vessels is infiltrated by inflammatory cells. This may spread to involve surrounding structures, leading to cellulitis or an abscess.

Lymphedema is an accumulation of interstitial fluid caused by obstruction of the draining lymphatics. The edema may be pitting initially. This may be caused by:

- Recurrent cellulitis.
- Malignancy.
- Surgical resection of lymph nodes.
- Radiotherapy causing fibrosis.
- Filariasis—nematode worm infection that leads to elephantiasis (gross enlargement of the skin and connective tissue).
- Postinflammatory thrombosis leading to scarring.
- Congenital abnormal lymphatics.

If lymphedema is prolonged, fibrosis of the interstitium may occur, leading to skin thickening and permanent edema. The skin appears to take on an orange-peel appearance (*peau d'orange*). Associated ulcers and brawny hardening of the skin may also take place.

If the dilated obstructed lymphatics rupture, then chyle (lymph with digested fats) may accumulate in parts of the body cavity. Chylous ascites, chylothorax, and chylopericardium refer to the accumulation of chyle in the abdomen, thorax, and pericardium, respectively.

Neoplasms of the lymphatics
Lymphangioma
Lymphangiomas are benign tumors of the lymphatic capillaries. They are analogous to hemangiomas. There are two types: simple and cavernous.

Simple lymphangioma
Typically, a simple lymphangioma occurs on the head, neck, or axilla. It can also occur on the trunk and in viscera.

Simple lymphangiomas are cutaneous or pedunculated nodules made up of endothelium-lined spaces in a network. No blood cells are present.

Cavernous lymphangioma (cystic hygroma)
Cavernous masses are usually present in the neck or axilla in children. They are not encapsulated, and they are poorly defined and therefore difficult to resect. Cavernous lymphangiomas tend to recur. There are dilated cystic spaces lined by endothelium.

Lymphangiosarcoma
Lymphangiosarcoma is a rare malignant tumor of the lymphatics with a poor prognosis.

Prolonged lymphedema is usually associated with the condition.

The tumor comprises multiple confluent nodules of vascular channels lined with endothelium.

Therapeutic interventions in cardiovascular disease

Direct, nonpharmacologic interventions are to be considered when:

- There is a lesion that can be treated by an appropriate technique.
- General measures and medical treatment have failed to relieve the symptoms.
- The benefits from surgery outweigh the risk of the procedure.

Treatment for arrhythmia
DC shock (cardioversion therapy)
Cardioversion therapy is used to treat serious ventricular tachycardia and fibrillation. A defibrillator is used to give a shock to the heart through the skin. This should abolish the arrhythmia and allow the sinoatrial node to take back control of the heart's rhythm. Implantable cardioverter defibrillators (ICDs) are available that can be implanted into the body. These ICD devices detect any arrhythmia that may occur, and they give a small shock to return the rhythm to sinus rhythm. Triggered DC shock is the treatment of choice for broad QRS complex tachycardias. The shock must be delivered on the S wave of the electrocardiogram.

Pacemaker
This is often used in sick sinus syndrome in which there is disease of the sinus node (ischemia, infarction, or degeneration), leading to pauses in sinus node function or bradycardia. Pacemakers can be implanted into the body to control the heart rate. An electrode is placed in the right atrium and linked to a voltage generator. This artificial pacemaker is then set at a certain frequency such that it takes over the role of the sinoatrial node in generating cardiac depolarization.

When there is heart block, a ventricular electrode is used. Heart block with intact atrial function requires a dual pacemaker.

Treatment for angina
Balloon angioplasty

Balloon angioplasty (percutaneous transluminal coronary angioplasty [PTCA]) uses information gained from a coronary angiogram, which shows the state of the coronary vasculature. It is usually used for the treatment of isolated, proximal, noncalcified atheromatous plaques, but it can be used for multiple lesions, and it can be repeated.

The method involves the use of a balloon that is inflated in the stenosed artery to cause dilation. The balloon is inserted through the obstruction in the artery using X-ray fluoroscopy and then inflated with a contrast material. Multiple inflations of the balloon compress and crack the atheroma. This should reduce the obstruction.

Complications are:
- Acute coronary occlusion.
- Restenosis (occurs in 30% of cases in the first 6 months).

Outcome can be improved using a device called a stent—a metallic "scaffold"—that is introduced around the balloon catheter. Inflation of the balloon fixes the stent in position, reducing the risk of restenosis. Newer stents elute drugs that reduce thrombosis and further reduce the risk of restenosis.

Coronary artery bypass graft (CABG)

For left anterior descending (LAD) artery lesions, the left internal mammary artery is detached distally and anastomosed distal to the coronary artery stenosis. For other main coronary arteries, a vein is taken (usually from the leg), and this is used to bypass obstructions. It is usually attached from the aorta to the artery distal to the obstruction. Multiple obstructions can be dealt with by these methods. Considerable improvement is achieved from the surgery in about 90% of cases (Fig. 5.34).

Complications are:
- Mortality (about 1%).
- Slow occlusion of the grafts.

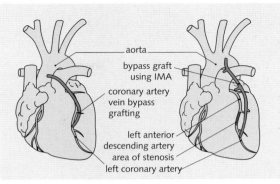

Fig. 5.34 Coronary artery bypass graft using a leg vein and left internal mammary artery (IMA) (redrawn from *Critical Care Nursing: Diagnosis and Management*, 2nd ed. by Thelan LA, St. Louis, Mosby, 1994).

Treatment for heart failure—heart transplantation

Heart transplantation has become the treatment of choice for severe, intractable heart failure in younger patients. Life expectancy would be about 6 months without radical intervention. The procedure requires the use of immunosuppressive therapy. With appropriate patient selection, the prognosis is good, with 1-year survival rates of 80% and 5-year survival rates of 70%. The quality of life in the majority of patients is dramatically improved.

Interventional procedures are generally more hazardous than nonintervention, but sometimes they can confer tremendous improvement in the patient, so that any increased risk is worth taking. For example, CABG has inherent risks in the operative procedure, but after successful completion, the risk of infarction is lowered compared with standard medical therapy.

- Define shock and its causes.
- Explain the clinical presentation of shock
- Describe the cardiovascular responses to hemorrhage.
- List the causes and risk factors of hypertension.
- Explain the differences between benign and malignant hypertension.
- Identify factors that can cause pulmonary hypertension.
- List the drugs that may be used to treat hypertension. Identify which combinations should be avoided and why.
- Describe how lipids are transported and metabolized.
- Identify the main hyperlipidemias.
- List the options available to treat hyperlipidemias.
- Explain the difference between arteriosclerosis and atherosclerosis.
- List the risk factors of atherosclerosis and explain how they can be reduced.
- Outline the series of pathogenic changes thought to lead to atheroma. Identify the cells and signals involved.
- Describe the complications of atherosclerosis.
- Explain why diabetes is a risk factor for atherosclerosis. Identify the other vascular changes associated with diabetes.
- Identify the main causes and types of aneurysms.
- Explain how you would differentiate between true and false aneurysms.
- Define aortic dissection and its possible complications.
- Identify the features of an abdominal aortic aneurysm.
- Identify the syndromes of ischemic heart disease.
- List the risk factors and etiology of ischemic heart disease.
- Explain the definition of angina and how is it classified.
- Explain the physiologic basis for the treatment of angina. List the drugs available for treatment.
- Explain how myocardial infarctions are classified and identify the pathogenic changes that lead to the different types.
- List the treatments available for myocardial infarction and explain how they work.
- Explain how sudden cardiac death results from ischemic heart disease.
- Explain how cardiac failure arises and how it presents.
- Explain how the body attempts to compensate for cardiac failure. Are these changes helpful?
- Identify the basis for the drug treatment of heart failure and how the different drugs contribute.
- List the forms of arrhythmias.
- Identify the mechanisms involved in causing arrhythmias.
- Explain how antiarrhythmic drugs can be classified. Identify the three general aims for drug treatment and the mechanisms involved in achieving these effects.
- List the valvular diseases and identify their sequelae.
- Identify the causes and complications of infective endocarditis.
- Describe the pathogenesis and features of the following diseases:
  - Dilated cardiomyopathy.
  - Hypertrophic cardiomyopathy.
  - Restrictive cardiomyopathy.
  - Myocarditis.
- Explain pericardial effusion and its causes.
- Identify the cause and results of cardiac tamponade.
- Describe the features of pericarditis.

- Describe the various classifications of the vasculitides.
- Identify the features of giant-cell arteritis and polyarteritis nodosa.
- Describe how the following conditions arise and how they present:
  - Atrial septal defect.
  - Ventricular septal defect.
  - Patent ductus arteriosus.
  - Tetralogy of Fallot.
  - Transposition of the great arteries.
  - Coarctation of the aorta.
- Identify the two important developmental anomalies of the vessels.
- List the effects of neoplastic disease on the cardiovascular system.
- Explain how a primary cardiac myxoma might present.
- List the types of hemangioma.
- Explain what telangiectasias are, and identify the different types.
- Describe the features of Kaposi's sarcoma in a patient with AIDS.
- List the risk factors for varicose veins. Explain how they develop. Identify possible sequelae.
- Explain how deep vein thromboses occur and how they can be prevented.
- Explain lymphedema and lymphangitis and how they arise.
- List the nondrug treatments available for arrhythmia.
- Explain the uses, risks, and prognosis of angioplasty and bypass grafting.

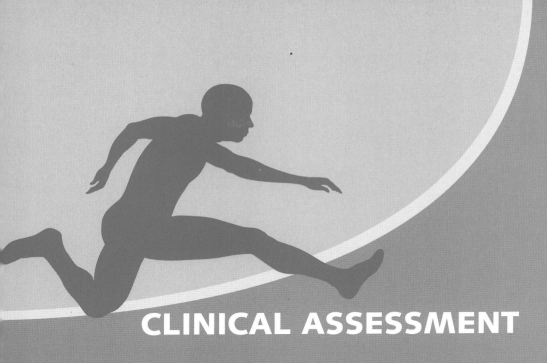

CLINICAL ASSESSMENT

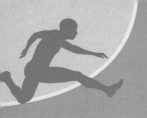

Common presenting complaints

Cardiovascular disease may present in a number of ways. Chest pain is the most obvious example, but shortness of breath or reduced exercise tolerance may be the first thing noticed by a patient. It should not be forgotten that some cardiovascular conditions may be asymptomatic, and these are diagnosed fortuitously when the patient is being examined for another complaint.

This chapter introduces the common presentations of cardiovascular disease and the differential diagnoses that they suggest.

Chest pain

When a patient presents with chest pain (Figs. 6.1 and 6.2), the following points must be investigated:
- Exact site, nature, and severity of pain.
- Onset.
- Duration.
- Radiation (e.g., to the arms).
- Precipitating factors (e.g., exercise).
- Relieving factors (e.g., rest).
- Associated features.

Angina

Angina is characterized by a constricting, tightening, or choking pain on exertion that is relieved by rest or nitroglycerin (NTG). The pain may radiate to the left arm and neck, and it may be exacerbated by emotion, large meals, or a cold wind.

Acute coronary syndromes

Acute coronary syndromes include unstable angina or myocardial infarction. They are characterized by spontaneous onset of continuous intense constricting or tightening pain at rest, which may be accompanied by sweating and vomiting. The patient may be very anxious and feel that he or she is about to die (sense of impending doom).

Acute pericarditis

Acute pericarditis is characteristically described as a sharp pain, usually localized to the left of the sternum. It varies in intensity with movement and respiration.

Dissecting aortic aneurysm

A patient with a dissecting aortic aneurysm may present with severe, sharp, tearing pain radiating to the back. The pulse may be slow and asymmetric.

Esophageal pain

Esophageal pain often mimics angina—it may be precipitated by exercise, and it may be relieved with NTG. It may be described as a burning pain with a history related to food intake or esophageal reflux.

Aortic stenosis and hypertrophic obstructive cardiomyopathy

These two conditions may also mimic angina.

Causes of central and peripheral chest pain	
Central pain	**Peripheral pain**

Cardiac
  Angina
  Myocardial infarction
  Pericarditis
  Mitral valve prolapse
	Respiratory
	  Pneumonia
	  Pneumothorax
	  Neoplasia
	  Tuberculosis
	  Connective tissue disorders

Aortic
  Dissecting aortic aneurysm
  Aortitis
	Chest wall disorders
	(cause pleuritic pain)
	  Rib fracture
	  Intercostal muscle injury

Pulmonary mediastinal
  Embolus
  Tracheitis
  Neoplasia
	Psychogenic
	  Anxiety

Esophageal
  Esophagitis (indigestion)
  Mallory-Weiss syndrome
	Other
	  Pulmonary embolus
	  Herpes zoster

Traumatic	
Psychogenic	

Fig. 6.1 Causes of central and peripheral chest pain.

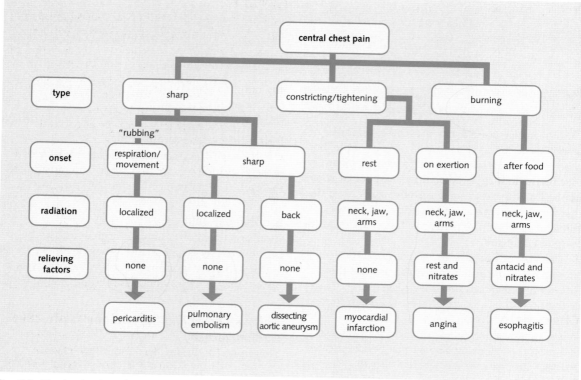

Fig. 6.2 Chest pain algorithm.

Dyspnea (shortness of breath)

How short of breath is the patient? Is the dyspnea brought on by exercise, or is the patient short of breath at rest? How much exercise brings it on (ask about dressing, climbing stairs, and walking). Dyspnea may be caused by:

- Heart failure if associated with orthopnea, paroxysmal nocturnal dyspnea (PND), or edema.
- Mitral stenosis.
- Shock.
- Respiratory causes (e.g., asthma, pulmonary embolism, pneumothorax).

Orthopnea

Orthopnea is shortness of breath while lying flat. It is a sign of left heart failure. Ask the patient, "Can you lie flat to sleep?" "Do you need to prop yourself up with pillows?" "How many?"

Algorithms for presenting complaints are only a general guide to establishing a diagnosis. Many complaints may strongly indicate a particular diagnosis, but the patient might have a different problem. For example, the patient may present with a burning central chest pain after eating. This may be indigestion, but it might be a mild myocardial infarction. Remember that medicine is not an exact science; you are always dealing in probability. The diagnosis will need to be confirmed with an investigation (e.g., measure levels of creatine kinase).

Paroxysmal nocturnal dyspnea

PND is a sudden shortness of breath at night, causing the patient to awaken. It is a sign of left heart failure and usually resolves when the patient sits on the side of the bed. Ask the patient, "Do you get attacks of breathlessness that wake you up at night?" and "How do you get over it?"

Edema

Ask the patient, "Have you noticed any swelling in your feet or ankles?" Peripheral edema is an indication of:

- Congestive cardiac failure—edema indicates the characteristic fluid retention of heart failure.
- Venous thrombosis.
- Lymphedema (caused by Nonne-Milroy lymphedema, radiotherapy, malignancy, or infection) if the edema is nonpitting (i.e., when you press the skin, no indentation remains).
- Other diseases (e.g., liver disease, nephrotic syndrome).

Hypertension

The World Health Organization (WHO) definition of hypertension is blood pressure higher than 140 mmHg systolic or 90 mmHg diastolic in the elderly. Blood pressure must be elevated on more than one examination for the patient to be diagnosed as hypertensive. If no organ damage is indicated, then blood pressure measurements should be taken over a long period of time before a diagnosis of hypertension is reached. Three consecutive readings of high blood pressure are usually required to confirm a diagnosis of hypertension. Mild hypertension is usually asymptomatic.

Secondary causes of hypertension are suggested by a specific history (e.g., sweating and tachycardia suggest pheochromocytoma).

Malignant hypertension often presents with:
- Visual impairment.
- Nausea and vomiting.
- Fits.
- Transient paralysis.
- Severe headaches.
- Impairment of consciousness.
- Symptoms of cardiac failure.
- Angina (due to atherosclerosis or high oxygen demand from hypertrophied myocardium).

Hypotension

Hypotension results if the systolic blood pressure falls below 80 mmHg. It often presents with the classic features of shock (e.g., tachycardia and cold, clammy skin). Hypotension can be caused by:

- Anaphylactic, cardiogenic, or septicemic shock.
- Volume depletion (hypovolemic shock)—hemorrhage, burns, gastrointestinal losses (vomiting or diarrhea), renal losses (diuretic therapy, nephropathy, diabetes mellitus).
- Drugs and drug overdose—opiates, barbiturates, amphetamines, antidepressants.

Commonly, postural hypotension results. This is a fall in blood pressure on standing (blood pressure should normally be maintained because of venoconstriction in the legs). Causes of postural hypotension include:
- Volume depletion.
- Autonomic failure (caused by diabetes mellitus or amyloidosis).
- Drugs that interfere with autonomic function (e.g., ganglion blockers or tricyclic antidepressants).
- Interference with peripheral venoconstriction by drugs (e.g., nitrates, calcium antagonists, α-blockers).
- Prolonged bed rest.

Heart murmurs

If a patient with heart murmurs is cyanotic, a shunt may be present. Note whether the murmur is causing the patient any distress.

Listen to the murmur in the auscultatory areas, and decide where the murmur is in relation to the cardiac cycle. Listen for intensity, any radiation, and any other associated sounds. Diastolic murmurs should be considered to be a serious sign. For more details and a differential diagnosis, see Chapter 7, p. 144.

Syncope (fainting)

Ask the patient whether he or she has recently fainted. The following points should be noted:
- Onset.
- Any loss of consciousness.
- Any warning (aura).
- Light-headedness or vertigo beforehand.
- Duration.
- Any memory loss.
- Any injuries sustained during the faint.
- Any incontinence.

Syncope can be caused by:
- Vasovagal attack—a powerful centrally mediated reflex, initiated by pain, powerful emotional stimulus, or sudden underperfusion of the brain (see Chapter 4, p. 73).
- Stokes-Adams attack—a transient arrhythmia that causes a loss of cardiac output. Usually, there is no warning (but possible palpitations). It causes pallor and an irregular or slow pulse.
- Aortic stenosis or intracardiac thrombus/tumor— produces a similar picture.
- Postural hypotension—occurs when suddenly standing.
- Carotid sinus syndrome—occurs in patients aged over 50 years while turning their head. Can be checked for by massaging one of the carotids while feeling for extreme bradycardia.
- Vertebrobasilar insufficiency—also occurs while turning the head.
- Respiratory causes—cough syncope or anxiety with hyperventilation.
- Other causes—hypoglycemia, elevated intracranial pressure, or alcohol/drug ingestion.

Abnormalities of heart rate and rhythm
Palpitations
Note any instances of palpitations. Ask the patient, "Do you ever notice your heart beat?" "Does it go really fast?" "Can you tap it out on the table for me?"

Palpitations may be caused by:
- Arrhythmias. A regularly irregular pulse indicates intermittent heart block or ectopic beats; an irregularly irregular pulse indicates atrial fibrillation.
- Anxiety.

Intermittent claudication
Intermittent claudication is an indication of peripheral vascular disease impeding arterial flow in the legs. You should ask the patient, "Do you get cramp-like pain in your legs while walking or at rest?" "How far can you walk?" "How long do you have to rest to allow the pain to go away?" "Can you walk the same distance after you've stopped?"

Elevated serum cholesterol and triglycerides
Hyperlipidemic patients might present with the following conditions or signs:
- Xanthoma (lipid deposits in a tendon).
- Xanthelasma or corneal arcus (lipid deposits in the cornea).
- Obesity.
- Hypertension.
- Pancreatitis.
- Diabetes mellitus.

Patients may also have a family history of lipid disorders or coronary heart disease. Secondary causes of hyperlipidemia must be excluded. These include:
- Hypothyroidism.
- Diabetes mellitus.
- Obesity.
- Renal impairment.
- Nephrotic syndrome.
- Liver dysfunction.
- Dysglobulinemia.
- Drugs (especially oral contraceptives, thiazides, corticosteroids).

A good method to use if you are stuck for a diagnosis is to employ a surgical sieve. This is a methodical approach to obtaining differential diagnoses by considering systems. Usually, the first approach is to consider congenital and acquired causes. The acquired causes are further subdivided. A mnemonic for this is **TIN CAN BED MD**:

T = trauma
I = infection
N = neoplasia
C = connective tissue disorders
A = arterial and venous disease
N = nervous system
B = blood disorders
E = endocrine
D = drugs
M = metabolic disorders
D = deficiency

- What questions should you ask to fully characterize a patient's report of chest pain?
- What are the presenting features of angina, myocardial infarction, heart failure, and pericarditis? How do they differ?
- What are the differential diagnoses for a patient presenting with chest pain?
- What can cause dyspnea?
- What can cause edema?
- How would a patient present with severe malignant hypertension?
- How would a patient present with hypotension? What would cause this condition?
- What can cause syncope?
- What other symptoms may indicate cardiovascular disease?
- What signs or symptoms may indicate a hyperlipidemia?

7. History and Examination

Taking a history

Important points to remember when taking a history include observation, introduction, and communication. These are discussed in more detail next.

Observation

Have a look around the bed for clues about the patient's condition. (Are there inhalers on the bedside table? Are there walking aids in the room? Are there intravenous drips, oxygen bottles, or monitors?)

Make an initial assessment of the patient. (Is the patient in distress, finding it hard to breathe? How many pillows is the patient using?)

This assessment should continue and be updated throughout the interview.

Introduction

Always greet the patient and introduce yourself, explaining who you are and what you are about to do. Try to shake the patient's hand. This is not only normal politeness, but it also allows you to ascertain some of the motor functions of the patient's hand.

Ensure that the patient is comfortable at all times. Be prepared to halt the interview if circumstances warrant (e.g., the patient might want to go to the restroom, or lunch might arrive). Remember you can always come back later.

If there are relatives around, do not be afraid to ask them to leave to allow you to talk privately.

If there are other people with the patient while you are taking a history (this can be daunting initially), you can use them to corroborate or give a different view on the information presented. Sensitive questions can be reserved until the examination, when you will be alone with the patient.

Communication
Nonverbal communication

Sit down at a comfortable distance from the patient. Give the patient your full attention, and make only brief notes.

Listen to what the patient is saying, rather than just writing it down; you will then pick up on comments that can lead to further questions. This is harder than it sounds, because frequently you are concentrating so hard on trying to think of the next question that you do not hear a vital clue. Keep the conversation flowing by nodding at appropriate moments.

Verbal communication

Ask open-ended questions ("What was the pain like?") rather than leading ones ("Was it a crushing pain?").

Let patients answer questions in their own words, without interruption. You should be aiming to hold a conversation rather than performing an interrogation. If you feel that the patient is rambling, gently try to steer the conversation back with a direct question ("If I could just clarify, what the pain was like?").

Try not to use medical terms (e.g., for orthopnea, ask, "How many pillows do you need to get to sleep?").

If a patient says that he has a certain condition, ask him to explain what he understands it to be and how it affects him. Beware of terms like "gastric flu." What does the patient mean by this?

Overall, try to be friendly and confident, and attempt to make the patient feel at ease. Do not be too worried if you cannot reach a diagnosis right away, but try to think of what the problem could be.

Presenting complaint

The presenting complaint is a symptom felt by the patient and not a diagnosis.

There may be more than one complaint; if this is the case, number the symptoms and take a history for each complaint.

History of the presenting complaint

Generally, you need to find out the following information:
- Nature of the complaint.
- Site of the complaint.
- Extent of the deficit. How disabling is it?
- Onset. What time during the day? Which activities bring it on?
- Course. How does the symptom pattern vary? What is the frequency—is it intermittent or continuous?
- Duration. How long has it been there?
- Precipitating and relieving factors.
- Other relevant symptoms.
- Any previous treatment or investigations for this same complaint.

You should usually let the patient tell you the natural history of the complaint, but you should specifically ask about the following symptoms:
- Chest pain.
- Shortness of breath, orthopnea, and paroxysmal nocturnal dyspnea (PND).
- Edema.
- Palpitations.
- Syncope (fainting) or dizziness.
- Intermittent claudication.
- Other symptoms—any coldness, redness, or blueness of the extremities (symptoms of peripheral vascular disease); sweating; fever; appetite change, nausea, or vomiting (symptoms of heart failure or digitalis toxicity); tiredness (might be caused by heart failure or ischemia, or may be a consequence of treatment such as β-blockers).
- Smoking.

Past medical history

Ask the patient if he or she has any other medical problems. Then say, "I'm going to run through a list of conditions to make sure we don't miss anything."

Important past medical conditions to note include:
- Diabetes mellitus.
- Hypertension.
- Myocardial infarction.
- Stroke (cerebrovascular accident [CVA]).
- Angina.
- Arrhythmia.
- Peripheral vascular disease.
- Rheumatic fever.

- Intermittent claudication.
- Renal failure.

Previous operations to note include:
- Coronary artery bypass graft (CABG).
- Angioplasty.
- Pacemaker insertion.
- Vascular surgery.

Drug history

A note should be made of all prescription and over-the-counter medications that are currently being used. Aspects of the presenting complaint may be due to current therapy. Be aware that some herbal and alternative medications have pharmacologic effects or interactions (e.g., St. John's wort and digoxin).

Any allergies should be noted, especially those due to drugs. To establish whether a true anaphylactic reaction takes place, ask the patient what happens when he or she comes into contact with the substance.

Family history

Any relevant family history should be noted. Ask whether there is any incidence of the following diseases in close relatives:
- Diabetes mellitus.
- Myocardial infarction.
- CVA.
- Angina.
- Hypertension.
- Any hereditary disorder.

Find out the state of health of the patient's father, mother, siblings, and children. If they have died, ask what they died of and at what age, but remember to be sensitive.

Social history

Inquire into the patient's marital status and children. Note the patient's present living conditions and any problems that these may cause (e.g., Are there many steps that the patient cannot negotiate?). Lifestyle, including diet and exercise, should be elicited:
- If the patient smokes, find out how many cigarettes per day and for how many years.
- How much alcohol is consumed? How often? It is notoriously difficult to get an accurate history of alcohol consumption: often, you must ask questions like, "How long does a bottle of whisky last you?"

- Has the patient ever taken any illicit drugs?
- Ask if the patient has traveled abroad recently.

You might also need to ask about sexual practices.

Occupational history

A careful occupational history should not be neglected. Find out the patient's current and previous employment, with particular emphasis on levels of stress and industrial exposure to chemicals or physical agents. Be aware that patients may be worried about the consequences of their health on their job and that there are medicolegal implications with certain careers (e.g., commercial driver, pilot).

> If patients mention an unfamiliar procedure or treatment, don't be afraid to ask the patient why they think they received that treatment. This will also help you to give better explanations in the future.

Review of systems

This is a systematic review of the whole body in an attempt to elicit any other symptoms. Points to note are outlined below.

Respiratory system

Note the presence of any cough or sputum. This may indicate pulmonary edema, and it also may be a side effect of angiotensin-converting enzyme (ACE) inhibitors.

Gastrointestinal system

Epigastric pain might be caused by simple heartburn or by a myocardial infarction. Other abdominal pain might be caused by an aortic aneurysm (if it ruptures, there may be continuous abdominal pain) or ischemia of the mesenteric vessels.

Increased thirst, if associated with other signs, may indicate dehydration, possibly caused by mild hemorrhage or shock.

Genitourinary system

Causes of increased frequency of micturition and increased urine production include diabetes mellitus and diuretic therapy. Intermittent tachycardias may also be associated with increased urine production.

Nocturia (needing to micturate at night) may be caused by heart failure.

Musculoskeletal system

Joint pain can indicate a systemic disorder with cardiac effects (e.g., systemic lupus erythematosus).

Nervous system

A note should be made of:
- Any visual disturbances (e.g., amaurosis fugax—seeing curtains drawn across the eye).
- Temporary blindness (due to emboli reaching the retinal vessels and causing ischemia of the retina—these emboli can arise from atheromatous plaques).

Observation of the whole body

General appearance

Note the general appearance of the patient. Is the patient:
- Well or ill/distressed?
- Alert or confused?
- Happy or sad?
- Thin or overweight?

Color

Look at the skin. Note any evidence of:
- Pallor/anemia—pale skin.
- Cyanosis/shock—bluish tinge.

These may imply:
- Hypovolemia in cutaneous vessels.
- Peripheral vascular disease.
- Pulmonary to systemic shunting.
- Lung disease.
- Hemoglobinopathy.

Rash

Look at any rash. Note size, type—macula (flat) or papula (raised), color, surface, and reaction to pressure—does it blanch or not?

Gross abnormalities
Marfan syndrome

Marfan syndrome is usually an autosomal dominant inherited condition. Those with the syndrome show the following signs:
- Elongated and asymmetric face.
- Dislocation of the lens of the eye (ectopia lentis).

133

- High-arched palate.
- Tall, with lower half of body larger than the upper half. The arm span is usually longer than the height.
- Long, thin digits (arachnodactyly).

Degeneration of vessel media can lead to a dissecting aneurysm in the ascending aorta, which may rupture. An incompetent mitral valve may also result.

Down syndrome

Down syndrome is trisomy of chromosome 21. Those with the syndrome show the following signs:
- Flat face with slanting eyes and epicanthic folds.
- Small ears.
- Simian crease (single plantar crease on the palm).
- Short, stubby fingers.
- Hypotonia.

There is a variable level of mental retardation. Up to 50% of children with Down syndrome have a congenital heart defect; the most common is an atrioventricular septal defect, followed by a ventricular septal defect.

Turner's syndrome

In Turner's syndrome, the genotype is XO (female). Those with the syndrome show infantilism (appear childlike even when an adult), a webbed neck, short stature, cubitus valgus (increased carrying angle of elbow), and primary amenorrhea (no menstrual bleeding).

Intelligence is normal. Other features can include coarctation of the aorta and other left-sided heart defects and lymphedema of the legs.

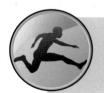

In an examination, if you are making a general inspection, make it obvious to the patient and the examiner.

The limbs

Fig. 7.1 gives details of hand examination.

There are few signs to note in the arms and forearms. However, the radial and brachial pulses must be assessed (see discussion to follow).

Fig. 7.2 gives details of examination of the lower limb.

Adopt a system for doing the examination. For example, always examine in the following order:
- Inspection, then palpation, percussion, and auscultation of each area that you are examining.
- Examine the hands, then the upper limbs, neck, face, chest, and abdomen; then examine the lower limbs.

Ensure that you use the same method when examining every patient with cardiovascular symptoms. In this way, you will not miss any signs.

Peripheral arterial pulses

Pulses should be checked as a matter of routine on all patients. Pulses on both sides of the body should be checked and compared. Blood pressure should be measured as outlined in Chapter 3, pp. 48–49.

Radial pulse

Palpate the radial pulse with the tips of the fingers, and gently compress the radial artery against the head of the radius. This pulse is often used to assess heart rate and rhythm. The pulse character is best assessed at the carotid. After locating the pulse, wait a while before counting the rate. The rate should be counted for about 30 seconds and then doubled to give a rate per minute. A normal pulse is between 60–100 beats per minute (bpm). Outside this range is bradycardia (<60 bpm) or tachycardia (>100 bpm). The rhythm may be regular or irregular; if it is irregular, note whether it is a repeating irregularity (regularly irregular) or completely irregular (irregularly irregular):
- Regular. Normal rhythm—remember sinus arrhythmia is normal (an increased rate may be noticed during inspiration).
- Regularly irregular. May be caused by ectopic systolic beats or second-degree heart block.

Examination of the hands			
Area	**Sign observed**	**Test performed**	**Diagnostic inference**
Nails	Clubbing (loss of the angle at the base of the nail) gap present / loss of angle normal / clubbed	Hold nails of both hands together and facing each other; if there is a gap, there is no clubbing	Infective endocarditis and cyanotic congenital heart disease Other causes: bronchial carcinoma, bronchial empyema/abscess, bronchiectasis, cystic fibrosis, fibrosing alveolitis, mesothelioma, Crohn's disease, cirrhosis, celiac disease, gastrointestinal lymphoma
	Splinter hemorrhages (small, linear, hemorrhages under the nail that are splinter-like)	—	Infective endocarditis; commonly found after trauma to the nail, especially in manual workers
Fingers	Nicotine stains	—	Smoking
	Osler's nodes (red, painful, transient swellings on pulp of fingers and toes)	—	Infective endocarditis
Palms	Janeway lesions (small, erythematous macules on the thenar and hypothenar eminences that blanch under pressure)	—	Infective endocarditis
Dorsum	Palmar xanthomas (lipid-like deposits in the skin creases)	—	Type III hyperlipidemia (increased intermediate density lipoproteins)
	Tendon xanthomas (yellow nodules over the extensor tendons)	—	Familial hypercholesterolemia

Fig. 7.1 Examination of the hands. Finger clubbing is an important sign of disease, and it should always be checked for. Clubbing is demonstrated by abnormal curvature of the nail, fluctuation of the nail bed, and loss of the angle between the nail bed and the nail itself.

- Irregularly irregular. Usually caused by atrial fibrillation or multiple ectopic beats.

The volume of the pulse should be assessed. A low-volume pulse implies decreased cardiac output. A high-volume pulse (described as bounding) may be caused by conditions including anemia, carbon dioxide retention, liver disease, or thyrotoxicosis.

Radioradial delay is delay of the left radial pulse compared with the right. This may be due to coarctation of the aorta proximal to the left subclavian artery.

Brachial pulse

Palpate just above the medial aspect of the antecubital fossa, and compress the brachial artery against the humerus. If you have trouble, palpate the tendon of biceps, and move your fingers medial to it. Use your left hand to measure the patient's right brachial pulse and the right hand to measure the left brachial pulse.

Carotid pulse

The carotid pulse should be palpated by pressing backward at the medial border of the

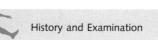

Examination of the limbs			
Area	**Sign observed**	**Test performed**	**Diagnostic inference**
Upper and lower limbs	Varicose veins (distended, tortuous veins; usually affects the saphenous veins)	Assess if they are hard (thrombosed) or tender (phlebitis) by palpation	Thrombophlebitis may indicate a deep vein occlusion; prolonged standing
Ankle	Edema	Press one finger in one place for 1 minute; see if the impression disappears quickly (normal) or not (pitting edema)	Fluid retention Congestive cardiac failure Lymphedema Deep vein occlusion Liver disease Nephrotic syndrome
Venous ulcer	Ulcers (breakdown of the skin that becomes very difficult to heal; venous: around medial malleolus; arterial: heel or toes) Xanthomas (itchy, yellow, eruptive nodules with red edge on extensor surfaces [e.g., buttocks]) Tendon xanthomas on extensor tendons	–	Deep vein occlusion Arterial disease Sickle cell anemia Diabetes mellitus vasculitides (polyarteritis nodosum) Squamous cell carcinoma skin lesion Hypertriglyceridemia Lipoprotein lipase deficiency Familial hypercholesterolemia
Leg	Problem with saphenofemoral junction valve	Trendelenburg test; lie patient down and raise leg; place two fingers 5 cm below femoral pulse (saphenofemoral junction); get patient to stand with fingers still in place; release fingers; if veins fill quickly, then valve is incompetent	Incompetent saphenofemoral junction valve

Fig. 7.2 Examination of the limbs.

sternocleidomastoid and lateral to the thyroid cartilage. The left thumb should be used to palpate the patient's right carotid pulse and the right thumb used for the left pulse. The two pulses should never be palpated at the same time, or you will risk restricting the cerebral blood supply. Make sure that there is no hypersensitivity of the carotid sinus that may cause a reflex bradycardia.

The carotid pulse should be used to assess the character of the pulse (Fig. 7.3). This is difficult, and there are also slight variations of normal. The important pulses to note are:

- Slow rising pulse. The pulse rises slowly to a peak and then falls slowly. It is of small volume. This may indicate aortic stenosis.
- Collapsing (water-hammer) pulse. There is a rapid rise to the pulse and then a rapid fall. It is usually found in aortic regurgitation. It may also be found in patent ductus arteriosus, ruptured sinus of Valsalva, or large arteriovenous communications.
- Bisferiens pulse. This is a combination of a slow rising and collapsing pulse. It is indicative of aortic stenosis and regurgitation (incompetence).
- Pulsus bigeminus. Ectopic beats occur after every normal beat but are too weak to be palpable, giving the appearance of a very slow pulse.
- Pulsus alternans. This is composed of alternating strong and weak pulses. It indicates severe left ventricular disease.
- Pulsus paradoxus. This is a pulse that is weaker or even disappears on inspiration. It can be a variation of normal. There is pulmonary venous distention caused by decreased intrathoracic pressure on inspiration. This leads to a fall in stroke volume

136

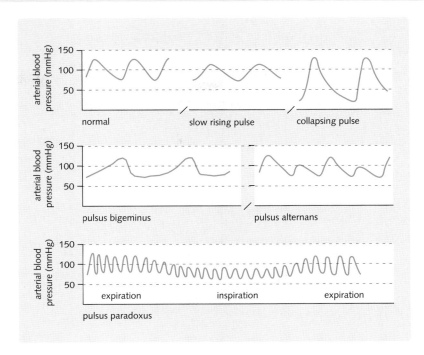

Fig. 7.3 Types of pulses. The various pulse waveforms that can result are shown here.

and, therefore, cardiac output. (When the heart rate increases to compensate, it gives rise to sinus arrhythmia.) If severe, this may indicate asthma, cardiac tamponade, or pericarditis.

You should also listen with the stethoscope diaphragm over the carotid pulse to detect any bruits (noise caused by turbulent blood flow). These may indicate that the arterial lumen has been narrowed by atheroma formation. Note, however, that the sound of turbulent flow can be heard far away from its source.

Popliteal pulse
The popliteal arteries can be found in the popliteal fossae behind the knee and are very hard to palpate. The thumbs of both hands should be rested on either side of the patella, and the fingertips should be placed deep into the popliteal fossa. The popliteals are best palpated with the knees flexed at about 120 degrees.

Posterior tibial pulse
The posterior tibial pulse is palpated about 1 cm behind the medial malleolus of the tibia with the patient's foot relaxed.

Dorsalis pedis pulse
The dorsalis pedis pulse is palpated against the tarsal bones on the dorsum of the foot.

Head and neck

Face
Fig. 7.4 describes the examination of the face.

Examining the fundus of the eye is a very hard skill to master. It takes great skill to do correctly and is best practiced under the guidance of a senior resident or attending physician.

Neck
Carotid pulses
The carotid pulse should be examined when taking all the other pulses.

Jugular venous pressure
The internal jugular vein will reflect the right atrial pressure. You must observe the maximum height of

137

Examination of the face			
Area	Sign observed	Test performed	Diagnostic inference
Eyes	Jaundice	Inspect the sclerae	Hepatitis; cirrhosis; hemolysis; biliary obstruction
	Cataracts (opacities in the lens)	–	Aging/injury; diabetes mellitus; hypercholesteremia
	Xanthelasma (lipid deposits above or below the eye)	–	Hypercholesterolemia
	Pallor	Inspect conjunctivae	Anemia
	Exophthalmos (protrusion of the eyeballs from their sockets)	–	Thyrotoxicosis
	Corneal arcus (crescenteric opacity in the periphery of the cornea)	–	Common in older adults; type IV hyperlipoproteinemia
	Lid lag (eyelid reacts much slower than eye gaze [i.e., when the patient looks up the eyelid is still drooped])	–	Hyperthyroidism
Pupils	Unequal	–	Unilateral nerve lesion; syphilis
	Irregular	–	Iritis; syphilis
	Hutchinson pupils (pupils on side of lesion constricts then widely dilates; then the other pupil does the same)	–	Increased unilateral intracranial pressure (e.g., intracerebral hemorrhage)
	Argyll-Robertson pupils (pupillary light reflex is absent but reacts to accommodation)	Pupillary light reflex	Syphilis; diabetes mellitus
Retina	Microaneurysm (small vascular leaks caused by capillary occlusion)	Fundoscopy using ophthalmoscope	Diabetes mellitus
	Hard exudates (yellow lipid deposits in the retina)	–	Diabetes mellitus
	Cotton-wool spots (white exudate around the macula)	–	Hypertension; arterial occlusion
	Flame-shaped hemorrhages (hemorrhage around optic disc spreading outwards)	–	Hypertension
	Retinal arteriosclerosis (copper-wire appearance of tortuous arterial vessels; nipping/indentation of veins as they cross arteries; white plaques on arteries)	–	Hypertension; general process associated with aging
	Papilledema (swelling of the optic nerve head caused by raised intracranial pressure)	–	Malignant hypertension; chronic meningitis; brain tumor or abscess; subdural hematoma
	Roth's spots	–	Infective endocarditis
Skin	Malar flush (peripheral cyanosis on cheeks)	–	Mitral stenosis
Lips	Peripheral cyanosis (bluish or purple tinge to lips)	(Unreliable sign of central cyanosis; therefore, also check the tongue)	–
Tongue	Central cyanosis	–	Pulmonary-systemic shunting; lung disease; hemoglobinopathy
Palate	High-arched	–	Marfan syndrome

Fig. 7.4 Examination of the face. Generally, this is restricted to inspection unless other systems are also being assessed.

the jugular venous pressure (JVP) and the character of the venous pulse as follows:
1. Place the patient at a 45-degree angle, with the neck supported to relax the neck muscles. You may need to turn the patient's neck laterally.
2. Observe the junction of the sternocleidomastoid with the clavicle, and then look up along the route of the jugular veins to determine if you can see any visible pulsations.

3. Try palpating the pulse. If you can feel it, then the pulse is probably from the carotid artery. Venous pulses are almost impossible to feel in a normal individual. Furthermore, the venous pulse is usually complex, with a dominant inward wave, whereas the arterial pulse is usually a simple dominant outward wave. The jugular venous pressure also decreases with inspiration.
4. Estimate the vertical height of the pulse from the manubriosternal angle.

The external jugular vein is often easier to see, because it is lateral to the sternocleidomastoid and more superficial. However, it is an unreliable indicator of central venous pressure. It contains valves and moves through many fascial planes, and so it is affected by compression from structures in the neck (Fig. 7.5).

A raised jugular venous pressure is usually indicative of:

- Heart failure.
- Superior vena cava obstruction (this also abolishes any pulsations).
- Increased blood volume (e.g., pregnancy, acute nephritis, excessive fluid therapy).

If the jugular venous pressure rises on inspiration (Kussmaul's sign), then consider:

- Constrictive pericarditis.
- Cardiac tamponade.

If the jugular venous pressure is normal, variation in the venous pressure waveform should be observed with the patient lying flat (Fig. 7.6).

If the jugular venous pulse is not visible, you may attempt to elicit hepatojugular reflux. This involves pushing on the liver, which should raise venous pressure and cause the jugular venous pressure to rise. You should place your hand on the right upper quadrant of the abdomen just below the ribs and push down into the abdomen and up under the ribcage, which will compress the liver against the diaphragm. The jugular venous pulse may then become visible. If the jugular venous pressure was originally so raised that it was not visible in the neck (i.e., the venous pulse was in the jaw), then this maneuver will not elicit any hange.

The jugular venous pulse is hard to see in healthy individuals, but when it is raised, it is usually very easy to see. Make sure that you see as many patients with this sign as possible, because it is highly diagnostic of raised venous pressure.

Auscultation

Remember to listen over the carotid vessels—see above.

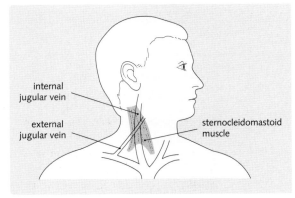

Fig. 7.5 The course of the internal and external jugular veins.

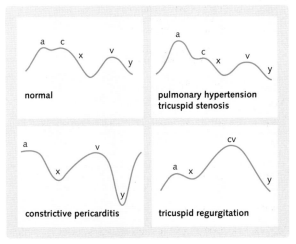

Fig. 7.6 The jugular venous pressure waveform in disease (a, a wave—produced by atrial systole; c, c wave—caused by transmission of increasing right ventricular pressure before closure of the tricuspid valve; v, v wave—develops as right atrium fills during ventricular systole; x, x descent—occurs at end of atrial contraction; y, y descent—follows the v wave on opening of the tricuspid valve).

Thorax

Inspection
Fig. 7.7 describes inspection of the thorax.

Palpation
Fig. 7.8 describes palpation of the thorax. Palpation is usually performed with the patient lying at 45 degrees. Fig. 7.9 shows the normal position of the apex beat.

If you cannot palpate the apex beat with the patient at 45 degrees, try turning him or her to the left-hand side. This should make the apex palpable in the midaxillary line.

Percussion
Percussion can be useful. Percuss over the position of the heart, and define the area of cardiac dullness A normal area of cardiac dullness does not reveal much. However, an increased area of cardiac dullness indicates cardiac enlargement or pericardial effusion.

A reduced area of cardiac dullness may indicate lung overinflation.

Auscultation
The stethoscope has two ends—the bell and the diaphragm (this is the larger, flatter end). The diaphragm is better for listening to higher-pitched sounds; therefore, it is best for hearing:
- First and second heart sounds.
- Systolic murmurs.
- Aortic diastolic murmurs (aortic incompetence).
- Opening snap of valves.

The bell of the stethoscope is best for low-pitched sounds. The bell should not be placed too tightly to the skin, because it will then function as a diaphragm. It is used to hear:
- Third and fourth heart sounds.
- Mitral diastolic sounds (mitral stenosis).

There are certain areas where auscultation should be performed (Fig. 7.10); these are the areas where murmurs from heart valves are best heard:
- Mitral area (and axilla if murmur present).
- Tricuspid area.
- Aortic area (and neck if murmur present).
- Pulmonary area.
- The back.

Inspection of the thorax		
Sign observed	**Test performed**	**Diagnostic inference**
Chest deformity	See *Crash Course: Respiratory System*	Bear the deformity in mind when assessing other factors (e.g., apex beat)
Scars	Sternotomy—midine scar in line with the sternum indicating that the thoracic cavity has been opened	Sternum has been cut for surgery on the heart or esophagus
	Thoracotomy—operative scar on the thorax	Sternum has been cut for surgery on the heart or esophagus
Masses	Lump in the left subcostal region	Pacemaker
Pulsations	Cardiac impulse; the apex beat can sometimes be seen; usually it is in the fifth intercostal space and in the midclavicular line (see Fig. 7.9)	Normal; If displaced, it can indicate left ventricular hypertrophy
Rarer pulsations	Diffuse pulsation not timed with apex beat	Left ventricular aneurysm
	Pulsation to the left of sternum	Aneurysm of the descending aorta
	Suprasternal notch pulsation	Aneurysm of the ascending aorta
	Pulsation to the right of sternum	Aneurysm of the ascending aorta
	Pulsation over scapula	Coarctation of aorta

Fig. 7.7 Inspection of the thorax.

Palpation of the thorax		
Signs observed	Test performed	Diagnostic inference
Position of apex beat (see Fig.7.9)	Place hand across the chest and feel with the tips of your fingers for the lateral edge of the pulsating apex	–
–	If the apex beat is not palpable, turn the patient on to the left side and then palpate in the anterior axillary line	–
Prominent apex beat	–	Left ventricular hypertrophy
Displaced apex beat medially	–	Lung collapse; lung fibrosis
Displaced apex beat laterally; apex beat more lateral	–	Left ventricular enlargement; pleural effusion; pneumothorax
Thrusting, displaced apex beat forceful and lateral, downward movement of apex	–	Volume overload—mitral/aortic incompetence
Sustained apex beat forceful and sustained impulse, which is not displaced	–	Pressure overload: aortic stenosis, hypertension; left ventricular hypertrophy
Failed detection of apex beat	–	Obesity, obstructed airways disease overinflated; pleural effusion; pericardial effusion; dextrocardia (very rare)
Parasternal heave pulse—left base of sternum	Palpate precordium	Right ventricular hypertrophy
Other pulsations noted on observation (see above)	–	–
Tapping apex beat, palpable first heart sound	–	Mitral stenosis
Palpable second heart sound	–	Systemic or pulmonary hypertension
Thrills	Palpable murmurs, which feel like the purring of a cat	–
Systolic thrills in aortic area	–	Aortic stenosis
Systolic thrill at apex	–	Mitral regurgitation
Diastolic thrill	–	Mitral stenosis; aortic regurgitation (uncommon)

Fig. 7.8 Palpation of the thorax.

Also use the diaphragm to auscultate the lungs from the patient's back to check for signs of pulmonary edema (see *Crash Course: Respiratory System*). Check for signs of lumbosacral edema.

Normal heart sounds

Many sounds can be heard with the stethoscope. Try to concentrate on hearing the heart sounds first (Fig. 7.11). There should be a sort of repetitive "lupp-dubb." Auscultating while palpating the

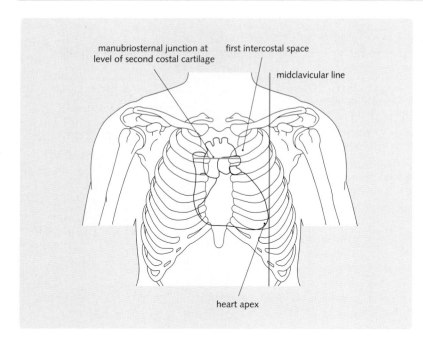

Fig. 7.9 Position of the apex beat. The apex beat is the position most inferior and farthest lateral that the cardiac impulse can be felt. As a guide to identifying intercostal spaces, the second rib lies lateral to the manubriosternal angle; the second intercostal space is below this rib. The lateral position can also be described relative to the anterior axillary line and the midaxillary line. The normal apex beat lies in the 5th intercostal space, midclavicular line.

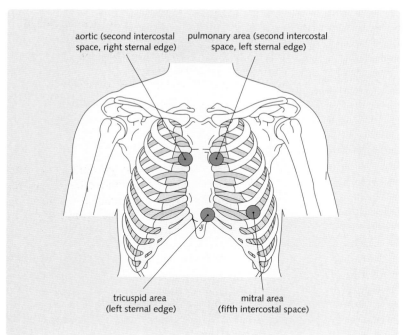

Fig. 7.10 Auscultatory areas. This shows where the valve sounds are best heard. These areas are not the surface markings of where the valves actually are (see Fig. 2.5).

carotid pulse will help to distinguish the heart sounds.

The first heart sound (S_1) coincides with the onset of systole and, therefore, the pulse. It is caused by the closure of the mitral and tricuspid valves. S_1 may be labeled M_1T_1 to reflect its two sources. The second heart sound (S_2) coincides with the beginning of diastole, and it is from the closure of the aortic and pulmonary valves. The components of S_2 are labeled A_2P_2. P_2 is only usually heard in the pulmonary area unless it is very loud.

Occasionally, the heart sounds may be split, when one component of the sound occurs before the other. For example, if the mitral valve (M_1) closes before the tricuspid (T_1), then S_1 is two distinct sounds, and it is said to be split.

S_1 is usually just one sound, and it is very rarely split. Any splitting of S_1 must not be mistaken for an ejection click or even S_4 (the fourth heart sound).

S_2 is normally split on inspiration (Fig. 7.12), especially in the young. Inspiration delays right heart emptying because it causes an increased venous return. This means the pulmonary valve is open longer and therefore closes later. This can only be heard in the pulmonary area.

Abnormal heart sounds

The third and fourth heart sounds (S_3 and S_4, respectively) occur in diastole (Fig. 7.13), and they are caused by abnormal filling of the ventricle. S_3 is caused by passive filling in early diastole. S_4 is a consequence of atrial contraction, leading to an increased filling pressure.

S_3 is sometimes heard in healthy, young adults (younger than 35 years) and in pregnant women. Otherwise, the presence of S_3 indicates:

- Heart failure.
- Mitral regurgitation.
- Constrictive pericarditis (the high-pitched "pericardial knock").

The presence of S_4 indicates a ventricle with increased stiffness (e.g., due to aortic stenosis or hypertension).

Clicks can be heard when abnormal aortic (e.g., in aortic stenosis) or pulmonary valves open. They are termed "ejection systolic clicks," and they occur in early systole—it sounds as if the first heart sound is split. Similar sounds occur with abnormal mitral or tricuspid valves, where the sound is middiastolic and is termed an "opening snap." A prolapsed mitral valve causes midsystolic clicks.

Fig. 7.14 shows some variations of abnormal splitting in S_2.

Alterations in sound intensity can indicate disease—for example:

- S_1 is loud in mitral stenosis.
- S_1 is soft in mitral regurgitation and first-degree heart block.
- S_1 is variable in second-degree heart block and atrial fibrillation.
- A_2 is loud in systemic hypertension.
- A_2 is soft in aortic stenosis.
- P_2 is loud in pulmonary hypertension.
- P_2 is soft in pulmonary stenosis.

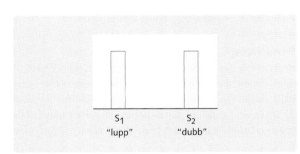

Fig. 7.11 Normal heart sound (S_1, first heart sound; S_2, second heart sound).

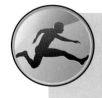

When listening to the heart, first concentrate on the heart sounds and establish that they are normal before attempting to listen to the murmurs.

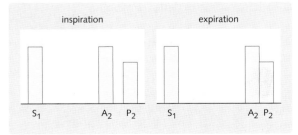

Fig. 7.12 Splitting of the second heart sound. S_2 may show physiologic splitting into A_2 and P_2.

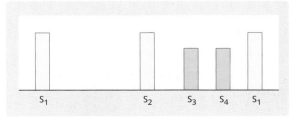

Fig. 7.13 The third and fourth heart sounds. The third heart sound creates a triple rhythm; the fourth heart sound is usually heard just before S_1 ("da-lupp-dubb").

Murmurs

Murmurs are caused by turbulent blood flow at a valve or an abnormal communication within the heart. It is customary to note the intensity of the murmur as a number out of 6 (e.g., 5/6 is a very loud murmur), but the size of a defect usually is inversely correlated with the loudness of a murmur. Not all murmurs are caused by disorders of the heart. These innocent murmurs are called flow murmurs, which typically:

- Are soft, early systolic murmurs.
- Have a musical or grunting component.
- Do not have a palpable thrill.
- Occur in the young or the elderly.
- Occur in conditions with increased blood flow (e.g., anemia, thyrotoxicosis, hypertension, pregnancy).

Murmurs are classified according to when they are heard (i.e., systolic, diastolic, or continuous) (Fig. 7.15).

Systolic murmurs are further classified into ejection (mid) systolic (intensity builds to a peak and then subsides before S_2) or pansystolic (same intensity throughout systole right up to S_2).

Murmurs are sometimes very difficult to hear when you are first starting out; it is best to try to differentiate whether the murmur is systolic or diastolic—it is most likely to be systolic. Then, try to differentiate between ejection systolic and pansystolic.

Even experts have difficulty in distinguishing some murmurs. Take every opportunity to hear as many normal hearts and obvious murmurs as possible.

In examinations in which you are asked to examine the cardiovascular system, first concentrate on the chest and then inform the examiner that you would also like to examine the abdomen. Usually, the examiner will say that there is no abnormality there and not to waste your valuable time doing this examination. However, you should take every opportunity to examine any patient fully, especially during your training.

Abdomen

Inspection

Fig. 7.16 describes inspection of the abdomen for scars and skin lesions, and Fig. 7.17 shows how to tell the direction of venous flow.

Palpation

Fig. 7.18 describes palpation of the abdomen.

Percussion

Percussion can be used to outline the liver. If the liver edge cannot be felt, then percuss over the right side.

If there is dullness throughout, the liver may be so enlarged that it occupies the whole area.

Auscultation

Auscultate over the abdomen, listening for bowel sounds.

If you suspect an abdominal aortic aneurysm, then auscultate over it to detect any bruits.

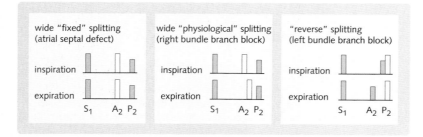

Fig. 7.14 Variations in the second heart sound. "Fixed splitting" occurs when the second heart sound is split, regardless of respiratory movements; "physiologic splitting" refers to the normal splitting of S_2 with respiration, and "reverse splitting" occurs when the normal changes with respiration are reversed.

Classification of cardiac murmurs			
Timing	Cause	Best heard	Radiates
Systolic murmurs: Ejection systolic	Aortic stenosis Pulmonary stenosis	Aortic area Left sternal edge	Neck Loudest on inspiration
	Atrial septal defect Outflow tract obstruction	Left sternal edge –	– –
Pansystolic	Mitral regurgitation (blowing) Tricuspid regurgitation (low-pitched) Ventricular septal defect (loud and rough)	Apex Left sternal edge Left sternal edge	Axilla – –
Late systolic	Mitral valve prolapse Coarctation of aorta Hypertrophic obstructive cardiomyopathy	Apex Left sternal edge –	– – –
Diastolic murmurs: Middiastolic	Mitral stenosis (low rumbling) Tricuspid stenosis Austin Flint	Apex Left sternal edge Apex	Louder with exercise – –
Early diastolic	Aortic regurgitation (blowing, high-pitched) Pulmonary regurgitation Graham Steell in pulmonary hypertension	Left sternal edge Right sternal edge –	– – –
Continuous murmurs: Combined systolic and diastolic murmurs	Patent ductus arteriosus (machinery) Aortic stenosis and regurgitation	Left sternal edge Left sternal edge	– Neck
Venous hum	High venous flow especially in young children	Neck	Reduced while lying flat
	High mammary blood flow in pregnant women	–	–
Pericardial friction rub	Inflamed pericardium; scratching or crunching noise	–	Loudest in systole

Fig. 7.15 Types of cardiac murmurs.

Inspection of the abdomen for scars and skin lesions		
Sign observed	Test performed	Diagnostic inference
Dilated veins visible	Check direction of blood flow by pressing vein and watching direction of refilling (see Fig. 7.17)	If flow of blood is superior: inferior vena caval obstruction If blood flow is inferior: superior vena caval obstruction If blood flow is adulating from umbilicus: portal vein obstruction
Pulsations in the epigastric region	–	Abdominal aortic aneurysm; visible peristalsis

Fig. 7.16 Inspection of the abdomen for scars and skin lesions.

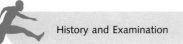

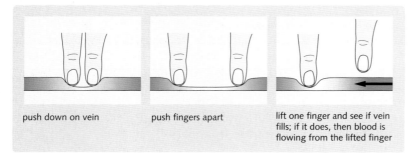

push down on vein   push fingers apart   lift one finger and see if vein fills; if it does, then blood is flowing from the lifted finger

Fig. 7.17 Assessing direction of venous flow.

Palpation of the abdomen		
Sign observed	**Test performed**	**Diagnostic inference**
Enlarged liver edge	Palpate right upper quadrant; feel liver edge by using the edge of your right hand and placing it deep; start low down and work your way up; ask the patient to breathe deeply	Right heart failure; infection; excessive alcohol use
Pulsatile liver edge	–	Tricuspid valve incompetence
Midline pulsatile mass	Palpate the epigastrium	Abdominal aortic aneurysrm

Fig. 7.18 Palpation of the abdomen.

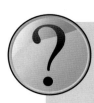

- What general points do you have to remember when taking a history?
- What are the specific points that should be covered about the presenting complaint?
- How would you take a history of a patient with a cardiovascular complaint? What specific questions would you ask?
- What signs can be seen by general inspection?
- How should you test for clubbing? What conditions give rise to finger clubbing?
- What are the signs of infective endocarditis?
- How would you inspect and palpate the limbs? What signs should you look for?
- Where should you palpate the peripheral pulses? How would you assess their rate and rhythm?
- What changes can occur in the pulse waveform?
- What signs of cardiovascular disease might be seen in an examination of the face?
- What changes in the retina might indicate cardiovascular disease?
- How should you view the jugular venous pulse? How does the jugular venous pressure change with disease?
- Which conditions can cause visible lesions on the chest?
- What disorders can change the apex beat?
- What are the normal heart sounds? Are there any normal variations?
- How do we classify abnormal heart sounds? How are the sounds caused? How do we describe their intensity and timing?
- What is the correct use of a stethoscope? When do you use the bell, and when do you use the diaphragm?
- Where are the auscultatory areas of the chest? What do abnormal sounds mean in the different areas?
- Which lesions of the abdomen may have a cardiovascular cause?
- How should you palpate the abdomen when looking for an enlarged liver or aneurysm? What might cause these disorders?

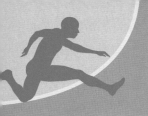

8. Investigations and Imaging

Investigation of cardiovascular function

Electrocardiography

The electrocardiogram (ECG) is a recording of the electrical activity of the heart, obtained by measuring the changes in electrical potential difference that occur on the skin. It is usually the first investigation used to diagnose arrhythmias and chest pain.

The electrical signal that activates contraction of the myocytes creates a wave of depolarization. As the wave of depolarization spreads through the ventricle, there will be, at any one moment, areas of the ventricle that have been excited and areas that have not yet been excited. In effect, there is a difference in potential between them: one area is negative in charge; the other is positive. These areas can be thought of as two electrical poles. This is the cardiac dipole (Fig. 8.1). This dipole depends on both the size of the charge (which depends on the amount of muscle excited) and the direction in which the

wave of depolarization is traveling. Recording electrodes are placed in certain positions on the body so that the cardiac dipole and other changes in potential can be measured in different directions.

Conventionally, the ECG is recorded using 12 leads (Fig. 8.2). Note that the term "lead" is used to denote the direction in which the potential is measured and not a physical electrode—only nine electrodes are used to produce the 12 leads. The additional three lead traces are produced using the "standard leads," which show the potential difference between specific pairs of unipolar leads. These leads allow us to view the electrical activity in both the frontal (I, II, III, aVR, aVL, and aVF) and transverse (V_1 to V_6) planes and in any direction in these planes.

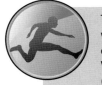

Think of depolarization as a wave on a pond that spreads out from a dropped stone. Where the muscle is narrow (e.g., the interventricular septum), imagine the wave being carried down a narrow channel.

Unipolar leads

Unipolar leads measure any positive potential difference directed toward their solitary electrode.
These include:
- aVL, aVR, and aVF—electrodes on both arms and the left leg. They view the heart in the frontal plane.
- Six electrodes labeled V_1 to V_6—these measure any potential changes in the transverse plane and are arranged around the left side of the chest.

Standard leads

The potential difference shown by these leads is conventionally measured from:

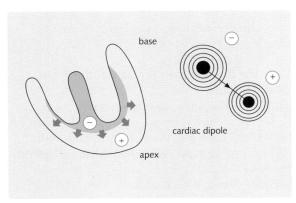

Fig. 8.1 The cardiac dipole. As the wave of depolarization travels from the atrioventricular (AV) node to the apex and base of the heart, it can be considered to move from an area of negative charge to an area of positive charge. The direction of the dipole at any time indicates how the wave of depolarization travels through the ventricle. (The area that has been excited is termed "negative" and the area to be excited is termed "positive." This reflects the changes in the charge in the extracellular space.)

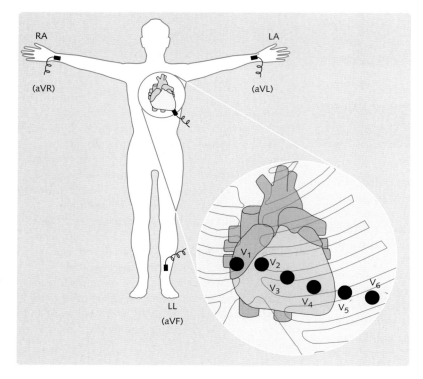

Fig. 8.2 Placement of electrocardiographic electrodes. The electrodes on the right arm (RA), left arm (LA), and left leg (LL) provide the electrocardiogram trace for the frontal leads (i.e., I, II, III, aVL, aVR, and aVF). The electrodes V_1–V_6 measure the electrocardiogram in the transverse plane.

- Lead I—right arm (aVR) to left arm (aVL); left arm positive.
- Lead II—right arm (aVR) to left leg (aVF); left leg positive.
- Lead III—left arm (aVL) to left leg (aVF); left leg positive.

These bipolar limb leads view the heart in the frontal plane. These three electrodes make up Einthoven's triangle around the heart (see below).

Remember that as the dipole has both charge (amplitude) and direction, the shape of the ECG varies, depending on the position of the recording electrode. The directions measured in the frontal plane and the associated changes in the ECG trace are shown in Fig. 8.3.

Normal electrocardiogram

The classic ECG trace is shown in Fig. 8.4. The elements of an ECG are:

- P wave—due to atrial depolarization and contraction.
- PR interval—due to conduction through the atrioventricular (AV) node (approximately 120 ms).

- QRS complex—due to ventricular depolarization (approximately 80 ms).
- QT interval—due to continuing ventricular muscle depolarization (approximately 300 ms).
- T wave—due to ventricular repolarization.

Note that the different components of the QRS complex are formally defined (Fig. 8.5).

Why the T wave is in the same direction as the R wave

The wave of depolarization travels from the AV node down to the apex and back up to the base of the heart. This is the cause of the R wave in the ECG. If repolarization of the heart then took place in the same direction, the T wave would be in the opposite direction to the R wave. However, repolarization actually takes place in a direction opposite the depolarization wave. Thus, the wave of repolarization is in the opposite direction to the wave of depolarization, and so the T wave is upright. This is a double negative: repolarization is negative depolarization, and it occurs in a negative direction; therefore, it appears as if it is positive.

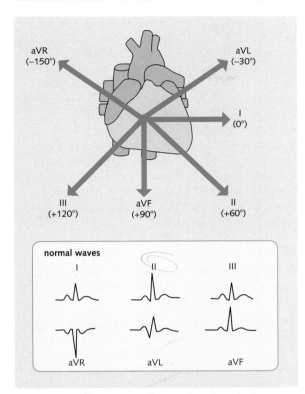

Fig. 8.3 Lead directions in the anterior plane (redrawn from *Clinical Examination*, 2nd ed. by Epstein O, Perkin D, de Bono D, Cookson J (eds), London, Mosby International, 1997).

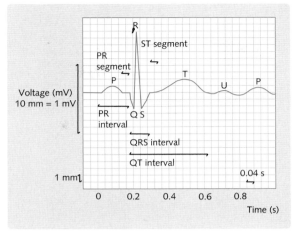

Fig. 8.4 Normal electrocardiogram.

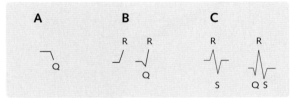

Fig. 8.5 Definitions of the ECG waves. A. If the wave following the P wave is negative, it is a Q wave. B. If a positive deflection follows the P wave, it is called an R wave, whether it is preceded by a Q wave or not. C. Any following negative deflection is known as an S wave, whether there has been a preceding Q wave or not. Abnormally large Q waves have an additional pathologic significance (see Fig. 8.12).

Cardiac axis

The average direction of the wave of depolarization is the electrical axis of the heart, referred to as the cardiac axis (Fig. 8.6). It must be established whether this is normal or not. There are three ways this can be established.

When the depolarization wave in the ventricles is moving toward a lead, then the R wave will be larger than the S wave in that lead. When the ventricular depolarization wave is moving away from a lead, then the S wave will be larger than the R wave in that lead. If the S wave and R wave are equal, then the depolarization is moving (on average) at right angles to that lead.

Therefore, to assess the axis, find the lead in the frontal plane with the greatest R wave. The cardiac axis is generally in this direction. Also, check that the lead that measures at right angles to this has an R and S wave that are approximately equal.

An alternative method is to count the maximum height of the QRS complex in leads I and aVF and plot

this point on a graph with the axes being I and aVF. Draw a line from the origin to this point. This reflects the axis of the heart (see Fig. 8.6). This is an analysis of vectors with amplitude and direction (as in the parallelogram of forces). A similar approach is used when drawing Einthoven's triangle (see Fig. 8.6).

The cardiac axis should be between +90 degrees and −30 degrees as shown in Fig. 8.3. Any deviation from this is abnormal and is termed right- or left-axis deviation.

Right-axis deviation (axis more than +90 degrees) is caused by:
• Right ventricular hypertrophy.
• Congenital heart disorders.

Left-axis deviation (axis less than −30 degrees) is caused by left ventricular hypertrophy.

151

and then spreads into the left and right ventricles (Fig. 8.7). Because the left ventricle is usually larger than the right, the average depolarization heads towards the left ventricle. This means that V_1 and V_2 will have a predominant S wave (i.e., negative deflection) and a small R wave, while V_5 and V_6 will have a predominant R wave (i.e., positive deflection) with a small S wave. The interventricular septum will be where there are equal positive and negative deflections (i.e., R and S waves). This steady increase in the size of the R wave is sometimes termed "R wave progression." If this is normal, then there is said to be good R-wave progression.

Rhythm disturbance
Rhythm disturbance is usually best assessed by looking at a long trace of lead II, which is often the closest lead to the cardiac axis.

Assessment of rate
The paper speed is usually 25 mm/s, which means that in 1 second the paper has moved by five large squares (i.e., 0.2 seconds per large square). Every small square represents 0.04 seconds. The rate can be measured in a variety of ways:

- Divide 300 by the number of large squares between QRS complexes. That will give you a rate in beats per minute.
- Find the time interval between R waves by multiplying the number of small squares by 0.04. Divide 60 seconds by this time interval to determine a rate.
- Find when an R wave lands on a large square. If the next R wave lands on the next large square, then the rate is 300 beats/min. If it lands on the square after that, then the rate is 150 beats/min, and so on. (see next bullet).
- If the interval between R waves is one large square, the rate is 300 beats/min; two large squares, 150 beats/min; three large squares, 100 beats/min; four large squares, 75 beats/min; five large squares, 60 beats/min; six large squares, 50 beats/min (i.e., divide 300 by the number of large squares between beats).

Assessment of rhythm
Note whether the rhythm is regular and whether every QRS complex is preceded by a P wave.

Note whether the PR interval is the same throughout. If the rhythm is irregular, is it irregularly irregular or regularly irregular?

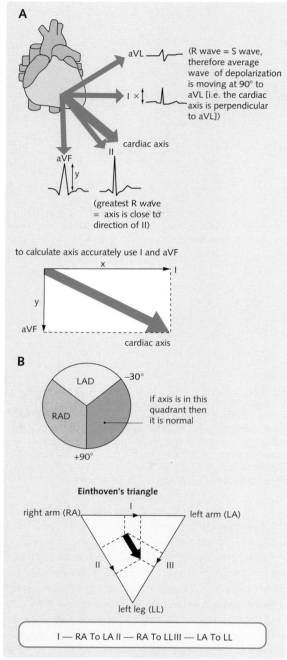

Fig. 8.6 A. Normal axis and the different methods to measure it. B. Einthoven's triangle (LAD, left axis deviation; RAD, right axis deviation).

Anterior chest leads (V_1–V_6)
The anterior chest leads monitor the chest in the horizontal (or transverse) plane. The wave of depolarization in the ventricles starts in the septum

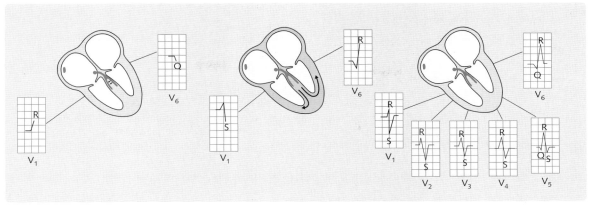

Fig. 8.7 The different anterior chest leads show different QRS traces due to the changing directions of the electrical activity. Lead V_4 is usually over the interventricular septum and therefore usually shows equal R and S waves. Note the changing relative heights of Q, R, and S waves between leads. The changing height of the R wave from V_1 to V_6 is known as "R-wave progression."

Arrhythmias

Heart block

Fig. 8.8 details the electrocardiographic appearance of the heart blocks.

Bundle branch block

Delay in the conduction system of the interventricular septum leads to widening of the QRS complexes (>0.12 seconds) (Fig. 8.9). Looking at leads V_1 and V_6 in right bundle branch block, there is:

- A second R wave (R') in V_1 and a deeper, wider S wave in V_6.
- The last part of the QRS in lead V_1 is negative. This reflects the delayed right ventricular depolarization.

This change can also be seen in lead I, where the last part of the QRS is negative due to the delayed right ventricular depolarization.

In left bundle branch block:

- There is a Q wave with an S wave in V_1.
- There is a notched R wave in V_6.
- The last part of the QRS in lead V_1 is positive. This reflects the delayed depolarization of the left ventricle.

Again, the delayed depolarization is also reflected in lead I, where the last section of the QRS shows a positive split peak.

Atrial and ventricular rhythm disturbances

Electrocardiographic appearances of atrial and ventricular rhythm disturbances are shown in Figs. 8.10 and 8.11.

Myocardial infarction

Electrocardiographic changes after myocardial infarction (Fig. 8.12) include:

- Within hours—ST elevation, and T wave lengthens and gets taller.
- Within 24 hours—T wave inversion, and ST elevation resolves.
- Within hours or days—abnormal large Q waves start to form and usually persist; T wave inversion may persist; ST segment returns to normal.

The leads in which these changes occur reflect the area of the heart affected:

- II, III, and aVF for an inferior infarct.
- V_1–V_4 for an anteroseptal infarct.
- V_4–V_6, I, and aVL for an anterolateral infarct.

In subendocardial infarction:

- There is T wave inversion.
- No Q waves form.

In true posterior infarct there is:

- A prominent R wave in V_2.
- ST depression.
- An upright T wave.

Electrocardiographic exercise test

An exercise or stress electrocardiogram is used to assess cardiac function in exercise. It is often used to diagnose angina. ST depression on an exercise electrocardiogram suggests myocardial ischemia. This may also be found in ventricular hypertrophy and abnormal ventricular conduction.

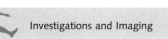

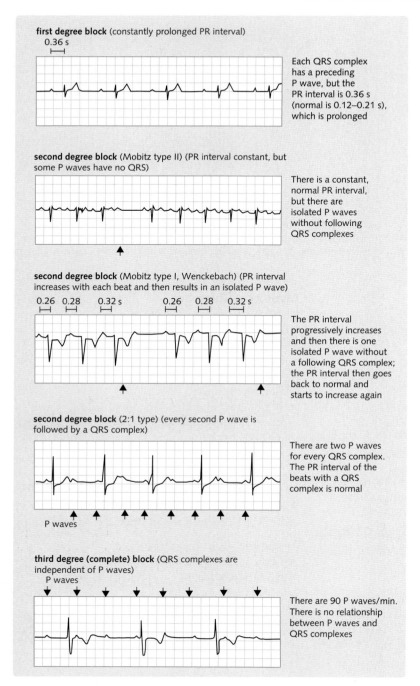

first degree block (constantly prolonged PR interval)

0.36 s

Each QRS complex has a preceding P wave, but the PR interval is 0.36 s (normal is 0.12–0.21 s), which is prolonged

second degree block (Mobitz type II) (PR interval constant, but some P waves have no QRS)

There is a constant, normal PR interval, but there are isolated P waves without following QRS complexes

second degree block (Mobitz type I, Wenckebach) (PR interval increases with each beat and then results in an isolated P wave)

0.26 0.28 0.32 s   0.26 0.28 0.32 s

The PR interval progressively increases and then there is one isolated P wave without a following QRS complex; the PR interval then goes back to normal and starts to increase again

second degree block (2:1 type) (every second P wave is followed by a QRS complex)

There are two P waves for every QRS complex. The PR interval of the beats with a QRS complex is normal

P waves

third degree (complete) block (QRS complexes are independent of P waves)

P waves

There are 90 P waves/min. There is no relationship between P waves and QRS complexes

Fig. 8.8 Classification of heart blocks. Note that only the large squares of the ECG are shown for clarity.

Other abnormalities

The following also affect the electrocardiogram:

- Digoxin—ST depression, T wave inversion.
- Hyperkalemia—tall T waves, wide QRS complexes, absent P waves.
- Hypokalemia—prolonged QT interval, small T waves, U waves (wave after T wave).
- Hypercalcemia—short QT interval.
- Hypocalcemia—long QT interval.

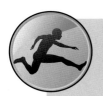

When assessing electrocardiograms, include the following information:
- Name, age, and sex of the patient.
- Date the electrocardiogram was taken.
- Rate.
- Rhythm.
- Axis.

Note any abnormalities and in which lead. Look at:
- P waves: width and height.
- PR interval.
- QRS complex: width and height.
- QT interval.
- ST segment.
- T waves: negative/positive and height.
- U waves.

Give a differential diagnosis.

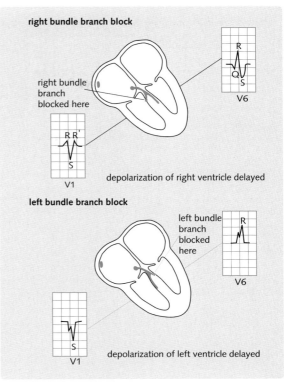

Fig. 8.9 Left and right bundle branch blocks. Disruption of the conduction system delays activation of ventricular muscle, producing a characteristic split peak in the ECG.

Echocardiography

Echocardiography is increasingly used as a diagnostic technique. The echoes of ultrasound waves are used to study the heart and its function. As the ultrasound beam travels through the body, echoes are produced at tissue interfaces, and they are reflected back. Echoes from tissues farthest from the transmitter take longest to return. In this way, a picture is built. Fluid generally shows up as black; tissues show up as white. Color is used to indicate blood flow on machines that combine echocardiography with Doppler ultrasonography (see following discussion).

Advantages of echocardiography for cardiovascular investigation include:
- Noninvasive, painless, and harmless.
- Can be used to study the motion of the heart and valves.
- Can be used to measure velocity of blood (using the Doppler shift phenomenon) and to estimate stenosis severity from acceleration of blood through a lesion.
- Can be used to measure cardiac chamber dimensions.

Disadvantages include the fact that the ribs and lungs do not allow ultrasound to pass through them, so special sites (or windows) must be used. Most imaging is still done through the anterior chest wall, but when necessary, an esophageal probe can be used for transesophageal (TOE) imaging.

Echocardiography is used to investigate:
- Valvular disease.
- Pericardial effusion.
- Aneurysms.
- Left ventricular size for a diagnosis of heart failure.

Doppler ultrasonography

This is used to measure flow in peripheral vessels. It uses ultrasound, in a way similar to that in echocardiography to map out the vessel highlighting any stenosis.

Red blood cells move relative to the ultrasound beam. They create a Doppler shift, which is a change

155

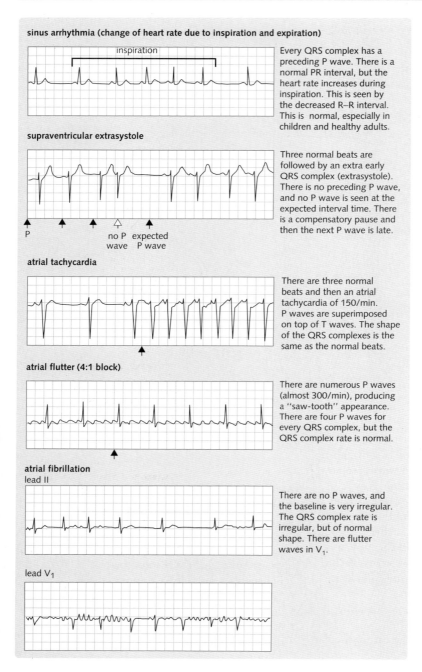

sinus arrhythmia (change of heart rate due to inspiration and expiration)

inspiration

Every QRS complex has a preceding P wave. There is a normal PR interval, but the heart rate increases during inspiration. This is seen by the decreased R–R interval. This is normal, especially in children and healthy adults.

supraventricular extrasystole

P   no P   expected
           wave   P wave

Three normal beats are followed by an extra early QRS complex (extrasystole). There is no preceding P wave, and no P wave is seen at the expected interval time. There is a compensatory pause and then the next P wave is late.

atrial tachycardia

There are three normal beats and then an atrial tachycardia of 150/min. P waves are superimposed on top of T waves. The shape of the QRS complexes is the same as the normal beats.

atrial flutter (4:1 block)

There are numerous P waves (almost 300/min), producing a "saw-tooth" appearance. There are four P waves for every QRS complex, but the QRS complex rate is normal.

atrial fibrillation
lead II

There are no P waves, and the baseline is very irregular. The QRS complex rate is irregular, but of normal shape. There are flutter waves in V_1.

lead V_1

Fig. 8.10 Atrial rhythm disturbances. These are also termed "supraventricular arrhythmias."

in the frequency of the ultrasound echo that returns to the transducer. The shift in frequency is directly proportional to the velocity of the blood.

Color can be used to differentiate blood flowing toward the probe from blood flowing away. It is commonly used to assess peripheral vessel function before angiography.

Cardiac catheterization

Originally performed to directly measure the pressures in the right heart, left ventricle, aorta, and pulmonary artery in patients with valvular disease, catheterization is now primarily used for angiography (see following discussion). Echocardiography is now the method of choice to assess valvular function.

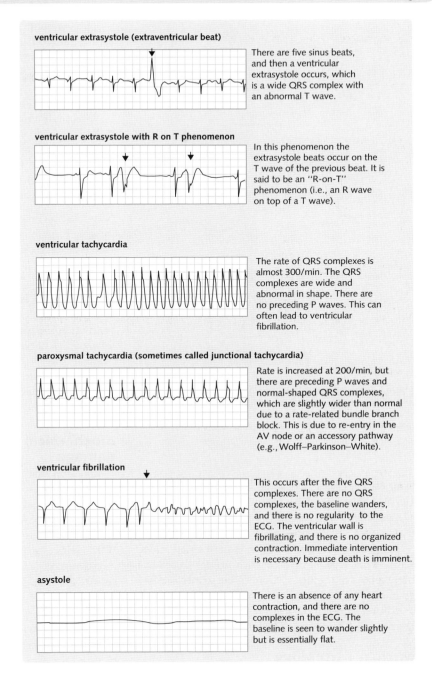

ventricular extrasystole (extraventricular beat)

There are five sinus beats, and then a ventricular extrasystole occurs, which is a wide QRS complex with an abnormal T wave.

ventricular extrasystole with R on T phenomenon

In this phenomenon the extrasystole beats occur on the T wave of the previous beat. It is said to be an "R-on-T" phenomenon (i.e., an R wave on top of a T wave).

ventricular tachycardia

The rate of QRS complexes is almost 300/min. The QRS complexes are wide and abnormal in shape. There are no preceding P waves. This can often lead to ventricular fibrillation.

paroxysmal tachycardia (sometimes called junctional tachycardia)

Rate is increased at 200/min, but there are preceding P waves and normal-shaped QRS complexes, which are slightly wider than normal due to a rate-related bundle branch block. This is due to re-entry in the AV node or an accessory pathway (e.g., Wolff–Parkinson–White).

ventricular fibrillation

This occurs after the five QRS complexes. There are no QRS complexes, the baseline wanders, and there is no regularity to the ECG. The ventricular wall is fibrillating, and there is no organized contraction. Immediate intervention is necessary because death is imminent.

asystole

There is an absence of any heart contraction, and there are no complexes in the ECG. The baseline is seen to wander slightly but is essentially flat.

Fig. 8.11 Ventricular rhythm disturbances.

A thin radiopaque catheter is introduced into the circulation and advanced toward the heart using occasional radiographs or fluoroscopy. The right heart is reached through a peripheral vein and by threading the catheter through the right atrium and into the right ventricle. The left heart is reached by a catheter entered through a peripheral artery and advanced through the aorta and the aortic valve into the left ventricle.

To produce an angiogram, the catheter is used to inject a radiopaque contrast medium into the heart or vessels. Angiograms are especially useful for viewing the coronary arteries for any stenosis. They are often performed before angioplasty or coronary

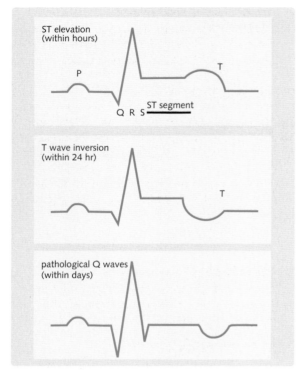

Fig. 8.12 ST elevation, T wave inversion, and Q waves after a myocardial infarction. Abnormal Q waves result from an electrode over an area of full thickness infarction.

artery bypass graft operations. Peripheral arteries can also be viewed with a similar process, with the catheter being guided to the arterial tree to be viewed.

If right heart catheterization is performed, blood samples can also be taken to measure levels of local metabolites in the heart. Congenital shunts can be estimated from measurements of oxygen saturation at different sites in the heart. Cardiac output can also be measured by thermodilution.

Nuclear cardiology

Nuclear cardiology is used to look at myocardial function, especially in ischemia. It uses radioisotopes, which emit radioactive particles that can be detected when they decay.

Different radioisotopes have different affinities for various tissues; for example, thallium-201 is taken up by healthy myocardium but not by ischemic myocardium, thereby mapping the ischemic area as a cold spot.

The technique can be used for subjects at rest and during exercise.

Commonly used methods in nuclear cardiology are:
- Thallium-201 imaging—to assess myocardial perfusion before and after exercise. It is used to detect ischemia and infarction.
- Radionuclide ventriculography—uses blood labeled with technetium-99m to assess ventricular structure and function. Ventricular diastolic and systolic volumes are measured, which can be used to calculate the ejection fraction.

Note that techniques using magnetic resonance imaging for similar testing are under development (see later discussion about magnetic resonance imaging).

Pulmonary investigation

The pulmonary circulation can be investigated using ventilation/perfusion (V/Q) tests, which check for mismatches between air entry and the supply of blood to the alveoli (fully described in *Crash Course: Respiratory System*). More invasive tests include pulmonary angiography, particularly when pulmonary emboli are suspected.

Biochemical markers of myocardial damage

Cellular enzymes and other intracellular proteins are released by necrotic tissue. Testing for the proteins specifically released from cardiac tissues can be a useful aid in confirming myocardial infarction (Fig. 8.13). The enzymes tested for include creatine kinase (CK), aspartate aminotransferase (AST), and lactate dehydrogenase (LDH), although tests for the classic cardiac enzymes have largely been replaced by measurement of troponin T (Tn-T) or troponin I (Tn-I), regulatory proteins on thin filaments, which leak from damaged myocytes. Tn-T levels peak 12–24 hours after myocardial injury but may remain elevated for over a week. Elevated plasma Tn-T is both very sensitive and very specific for cardiac damage, but episodes of reversible ischemia may also elevate plasma troponin levels. Current guidelines are that a peak plasma Tn-T between 0.1 and 0.2 ng/mL indicates unstable angina, with a peak plasma Tn-T > 0.2 ng/mL indicating myocardial infarction.

Myoglobin, a protein that aids the transport of oxygen in the cells, is also sometimes used. This peaks at 2–4 hours and may persist for several days.

Creatine kinase

Creatine kinase peaks within 24 hours of infarction and returns to normal within 2 days. It is also produced by skeletal muscle and brain, so the isoenzyme specific to myocardium (CK–MB) is usually measured. The level of enzyme released directly relates to the size of the infarction.

Creatine kinase levels can also be increased as a result of an intramuscular injection or the patient falling.

This enzyme is usually used to confirm a diagnosis of myocardial infarction.

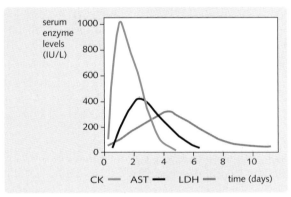

Fig. 8.13 Levels of classic cardiac enzymes after myocardial infarction (CK, creatine kinase; AST, aspartate aminotransferase; LDH, lactate dehydrogenase) (redrawn from *Color Atlas and Text of Clinical Medicine* by Forbes CD, Jackson WF, St. Louis, Mosby, 1993).

Aspartate aminotransferase

Aspartate aminotransferase peaks after 1–2 days, and it returns to normal within 3 days. It is also produced from liver, kidney, lungs, and red blood cells.

Lactate dehydrogenase

Lactate dehydrogenase peaks after 2–3 days and stays high for 1 week. It is also released from skeletal muscle, liver, and red blood cells. LDH-1—also known as hydroxybutyrate dehydrogenase (HBD)—is the most cardiospecific of the five isoenzymes of lactate dehydrogenase. Lactate dehydrogenase is often used for a retrospective diagnosis of myocardial infarction.

Routine investigations

Hematology

Fig. 8.14 outlines the tests that can be performed when assessing haematological problems in the cardiovascular system.

Clinical chemistry

Fig. 8.15 outlines the clinical chemistry tests that can be performed when assessing the cardiovascular system. Much biochemical data cannot be looked at individually (e.g., in dehydration there will probably be an increased concentration of sodium, potassium, chloride, and other substances). Usually, these tests

Normal values for clinical hematology			
Component	**Normal range**	**Change from normal**	**Reason**
Hemoglobin	Male: 13–17 g/dL	High	Polycythemia
	Female: 12–15 g/dL	Low	Anemia
Red blood cells	Male: 4.4–5.8 × 10^{12}/L	High	Polycythemia
	Female: 4.0–5.2 × 10^{12}/L	Low	Anemia
White blood cells	4–10 × 10^9/L	High	Infection, trauma, hemorrhage, inflammation, infarction
		Low	Infection, corticosteroid therapy
Platelet count	150–400 × 10^9/L	High	Thrombocythemia
		Low	Thrombocytopenia
Erythrocyte sedimentation rate (ESR)	Male: <age in years/2 Female: <(age in years) + 100/2	High: nonspecific indication of disease	Myocardial infarction, vasculitis, systemic lupus erythematosus, rheumatoid arthritis, malignancy

Fig. 8.14 Normal values for clinical hematology.

Normal values in clinical chemistry			
Substance analyzed	Normal range	Change from normal	Causes
Electrolytes: Urea	3.3–6.7 mmol/L	High	Renal failure
Creatinine	60–120 μmol/L	High	Renal failure
Na⁺	135–145 mmol/L	High Low	Dehydration hypereldosteronism Diuretics, aldosterone deficiency, water excess
K⁺	3.6–5.0 mmol/L	High or low	Can lead to anthythnins
Cl⁻	100–110 mmol/L	–	–
Ca²⁺	2.2–2.6 mmol/L	High Low	Malignancy, thiazide diuretics, thyrotoxicosis Renal failure, blood transfusion
HCO₃⁻	24–30 mmol/L	High Low	Metabolic/respiratory alkalosis Metabolic/respiratory acidosis
Glucose (fasting)	2.8–6.0 mmol/L	High	Impaired glucose tolerance
pO₂ (arterial)	11–15 kPa (85–106 mmHg)	Low	Respiratory failure Hyperventilation
pCO₂ (arterial)	4.5–6.0 kPa (35–46 mmHg)	Low High	Respiratory failure
Thyroid function: TSH T₄ T₃	0.3–0.6 mol/L 5–26 pmol/L 3–8.8 pmol/L	High TSH, low T₄, T₃ Low TSH, high T₄, T₃	Hypothyroidism Hyperthyroidism
Cholesterol: total	<5.2 mmol/L	High	Hypercholesterolemia (may be familial)
High-density lipoprotein	>1.2 mmol/L	Low	Predisposes to atherosclerosis
Low-density lipoprotein	<3.5 mmol/L	High	Hypercholesterolemia (may be familial)
Triglyceride (fasting)	0.4–1.8 mmol/L	High	Hyperlipidemia
Osmolality	280–295 mmol/L	High Low	Dehydration Water overload

Fig. 8.15 Normal values in clinical chemistry (T_3, tri-iodothyronine; T_4, thyroxine; TSH, thyroid-stimulating hormone).

are performed using blood, but urine can also be tested (e.g., for protein, glucose).

Microbiology

Any sample of the body can be sent for cell culture and sensitivity testing. The microbiology department will attempt to grow any microorganisms present (culture) and determine what antibiotics can be used in treatment (sensitivity).

Viral serology may help to diagnose acute myocarditis (coxsackievirus). Samples sent are usually blood or sputum. Blood is indicated for suspected cases of infective endocarditis (*Streptococcus viridans*) and rheumatic fever

(*Streptococcus pyogenes*). Sputum is indicated for suspected cases of tuberculosis (*Mycobacterium tuberculosis*).

Frequently, an abnormality in one lab test is not diagnostic of a condition. You must look at various factors to reach a definitive diagnosis. For example, a raised ESR and white cell count may indicate infection, but this can be confirmed only by a positive culture or serologic test.

Histopathology

Usually, samples sent for histopathologic diagnosis are biopsies of the lesion. It is most commonly used for the following:

- Vasculitis—polyarteritis nodosa, Wegener's granulomatosis, and Takayasu's arteritis.
- Cardiac tumors—atrial myxoma.
- Vascular tumors—hemangiomas.

Imaging of the cardiovascular system

Radiography
Plain radiography

Examples of plain chest radiographs are shown in Figs. 8.16–8.19.

Fig. 8.16 shows a normal posteroanterior (PA) chest radiograph. The width of the heart shadow is less than half of the transthoracic diameter. Note that it is only possible to comment on the heart size on the PA radiograph and not on an anteroposterior (AP) view.

A normal lateral chest radiograph is shown in Fig. 8.17. This is a useful view, especially if an abnormality is seen on the PA chest radiograph. It helps to localize any lesions. For example, left atrial enlargement is seen as a posterior projection indenting the esophagus. Fig. 8.18 shows an aneurysm of the left ventricle. Fig. 8.19 shows heart failure, with early pulmonary congestion.

Angiography

Fig. 8.20 shows examples of normal right and left pulmonary angiograms. An example of pulmonary embolism of the right and left lobe is shown in Fig. 8.21.

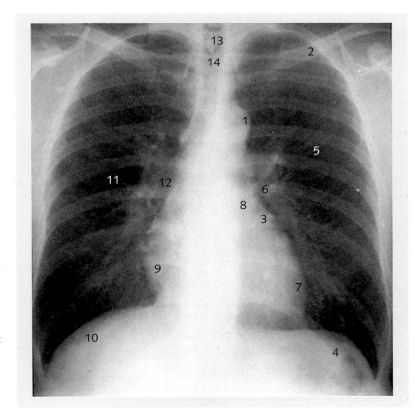

Fig. 8.16 Normal posteroanterior (PA) chest radiograph (1, arch of aorta/aortic knob; 2, clavicle; 3, left atrial appendage; 4, left dome of diaphragm; 5, left lung; 6, left hilum; 7, left ventricular border; 8, pulmonary trunk; 9, right atrial border; 10, right dome of diaphragm; 11, right lung; 12, right hilum; 13; spine of vertebrae; 14, trachea) (courtesy of Professor Dame M. Turner-Warwick, Dr. M. Hodson, Professor B. Corrin, and Dr. I. Kerr).

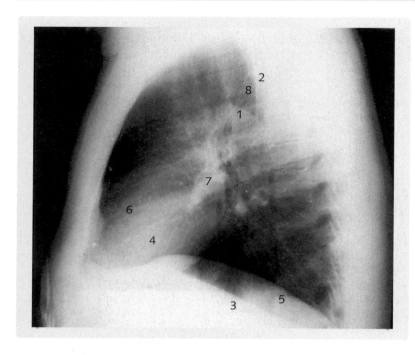

Fig. 8.17 Normal lateral chest radiograph (1, aortic arch; 2, anterior borders of scapulae; 3, left dome of diaphragm; 4, left ventricle; 5, right dome of diaphragm; 6, right ventricle; 7, left atrium; 8, trachea) (courtesy of Professor Dame M. Turner-Warwick, Dr. M. Hodson, Professor B. Corrin, and Dr. I. Kerr).

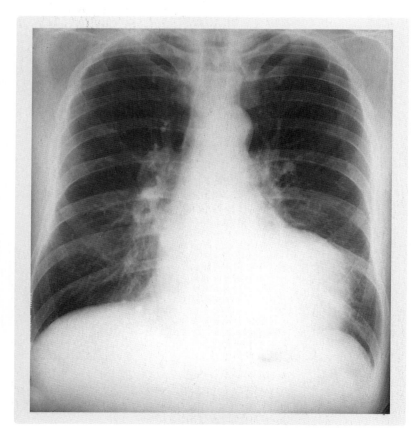

Fig. 8.18 Radiograph of an aneurysm of the left ventricle. This is a rare source of arterial embolism, which may occur some months after a myocardial infarct. Note the large heart shadow and how it occupies more than half of the transthoracic diameter. Contrast the normal appearance of the lung fields here with the congested fields in Fig. 8.19 (courtesy of Professor J.J.F. Belch, Mr. P.T. McCollum, Mr. P.A. Stonebridge, and Professor W.F. Walker).

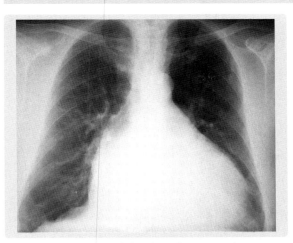

Fig. 8.19 Radiograph of the chest showing early pulmonary congestion. Note that the width of the heart shadow is greater than half the transthoracic diameter and that there are distended hila with increased lung markings. This indicates heart failure and pulmonary congestion (courtesy of Dr. A. Timmis and Dr. S. Brecker).

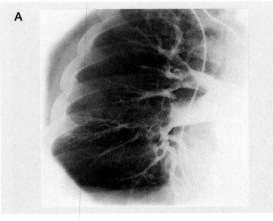

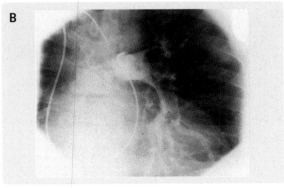

Fig. 8.21 Pulmonary angiograms showing pulmonary embolism of the right lung (A) and left lung (B). Contrast agent does not reach the distal part of the arterial tree, implying that there is some blockage (courtesy of Dr. A. Timmis and Dr. S. Brecker).

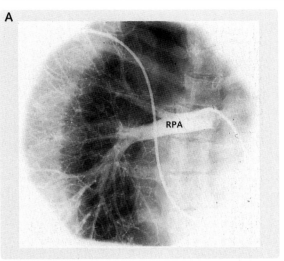

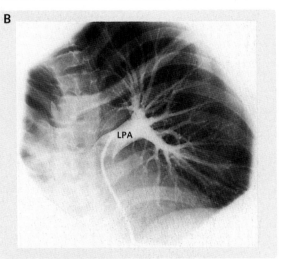

Fig. 8.20 Normal right (A) and left (B) pulmonary angiograms. The contrast agent highlights the entire arterial tree from the right and left pulmonary arteries (LPA, left pulmonary artery; RPA, right pulmonary artery) (courtesy of Dr. A. Timmis and Dr. S. Brecker).

Ultrasound
Echocardiography

A parasternal long axis view is shown in Fig. 8.22, and an intracardiac thrombus is shown in Fig. 8.23; mitral stenosis is shown in Fig. 8.24.

163

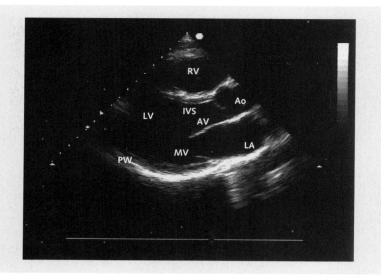

Fig. 8.22 Echocardiogram of the parasternal long axis view (diastolic frame) (Ao, aorta; AV, aortic valve; IVS, intraventricular septum; LA, left atrium; LV, left ventricle; MV, mitral valve; PW, posterior LV wall; RV, right ventricle) (courtesy of Dr. A. Timmis and Dr. S. Brecker).

 A good system for looking at radiographs includes all of the following information and questions:
- Name, age, and sex of patient.
- Date radiograph was taken.
- Is it AP (anteroposterior) or PA (posteroanterior)?
- Is it erect or supine?
- What is the penetration like (are the vertebral bodies just visible under the heart)?
- Is there any rotation (are the clavicles symmetric)?
- Describe any abnormalities in the:
  - Mediastinum.
  - Cardiac shadow.
  - Lung fields.
  - Ribs.
  - Diaphragm.
- Suggest a differential diagnosis.

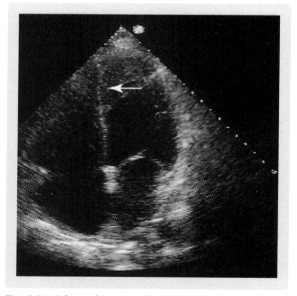

Fig. 8.23 Echocardiogram of an intracardiac thrombus. Here, the layered thrombus *(arrow)* is shown at the cardiac apex in relation to a previous myocardial infarct (courtesy of Dr. A. Timmis and Dr. S. Brecker).

Tomography
Computerized tomography (CT)
An example of an aortic aneurysm is shown in Fig. 8.25.

This imaging modality enables precise measurement of the size of the aneurysm. The whole body is imaged as slices or sections using radiographs. It can be used to produce a three-dimensional image, and it may also be used to perform angiography using radiopaque contrast medium.

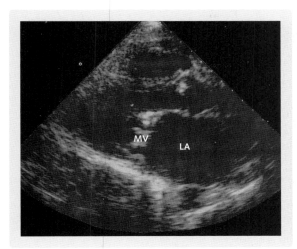

Fig. 8.24 Echocardiogram of mitral stenosis *(long axis)*. The mitral valve (MV) leaflets are densely thickened, and the left atrium (LA) is severely dilated (courtesy of Dr. A. Timmis and Dr. S. Brecker).

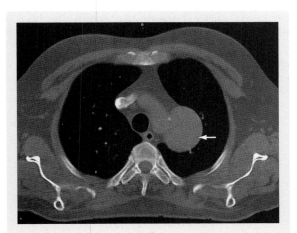

Fig. 8.25 CT of a thoracic aortic aneurysm. The scan shows a large aneurysm of the descending aortic arch *(arrow)* arising just after the left subclavian branch. This is the typical location for dissecting aortic aneurysms, although a dissection cannot be seen in this film (courtesy of Dr. A. Timmis and Dr. S. Brecker).

Magnetic resonance imaging (MRI)

MRI of the chest enables an accurate assessment to be made of the dimensions of the heart walls and lumen. Fig. 8.26 shows a normal coronal view of the chest, and Fig. 8.27 shows an extensive aortic dissection.

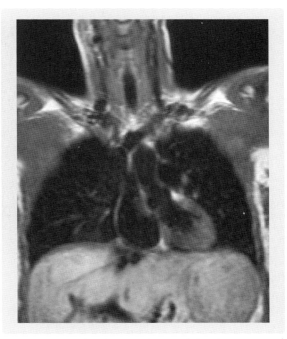

Fig. 8.26 Normal MRI coronal view of the chest (courtesy of Dr. A. Timmis and Dr. S. Brecker).

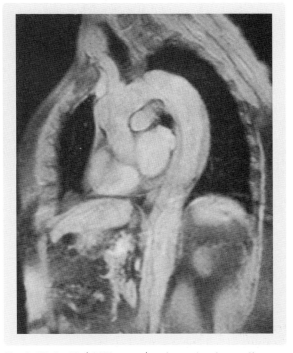

Fig. 8.27 Sagittal MRI scan showing extensive aortic dissection. Note how the descending aorta seems to have two lumens (double-barreled) (courtesy of Dr. A. Timmis and Dr. S. Brecker).

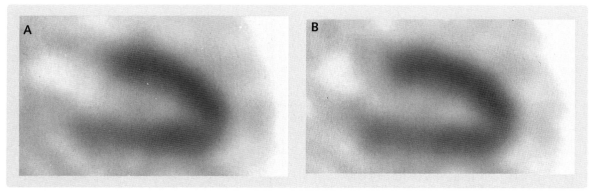

Fig. 8.28 Nuclear tomograms at rest (A) and during exercise (B) after injection of ^{99m}Tc-labeled MIBI, demonstrating myocardial perfusion. The example shown here is a vertical long axis view (courtesy of Dr. A. Timmis and Dr. S .Brecker).

MRI allows better visualization of soft tissue than CT. It is safer than CT, because it does not involve harmful radiation. MRI may also be set to show moving blood to produce an image similar to an angiogram. This has replaced conventional angiography for peripheral arteries, when MRI is available. Heart movement currently restricts the visualization of the coronary arteries to the large proximal vessels only.

The use of gadolinium as a contrast agent allows delineation of perfused myocardium during the first pass and of infarcted tissue 15–20 minutes later.

Nuclear imaging

Fig. 8.28 shows nuclear tomograms after injection of ^{99m}Tc-labeled methoxyisobutyl isonitrile (MIBI), demonstrating myocardial perfusion. Isotope is distributed homogeneously throughout the left ventricular myocardium, at rest and during exercise, reflecting normal myocardial perfusion.

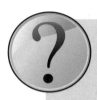

- What does the ECG measure?
- What is the cardiac dipole? How does it arise?
- What is the difference between a lead and an electrode? What are the two different kinds of lead?
- Where would you place electrocardiograph electrodes?
- Sketch a "typical" ECG trace, showing the normal wave and normal parameters.
- How do you determine the cardiac axis?
- How does the ECG trace change across the anterior chest leads? Do any have a special location? What can you learn from looking at the trace across all six leads?
- What are the major types of arrhythmia?
- How does the electrocardiogram change in these arrhythmias?
- What electrocardiographic changes occur in myocardial infarction?
- When would you use echocardiography? What would you be looking for?
- What is the major role of cardiac catheterization?
- What is the "Doppler shift"? How is it useful?
- How do cardiac enzyme levels in blood change after a myocardial infarction?
- What are the normal values for hemoglobin, white blood cells, and ESR?
- What decreases hemoglobin levels? What can increase the ESR?
- Which electrolytes are usually measured? What are their normal levels?
- How would you view a plain radiograph?
- What is the basis for thallium imaging in nuclear cardiology?
- How would you interpret other images of the cardiovascular system?

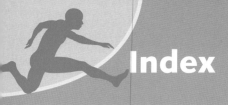

Index

Page numbers for figures are indicated by bold type.

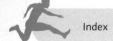

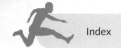

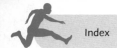

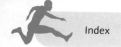

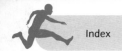

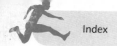